Coping with the Emotional Impact of Cancer

D1533885

Also by Neil Fiore, Ph.D.

Conquering Test Anxiety co-authored with Susan C. Pescar
(Warner Books, 1987)

*Awaken Your Strongest Self: Break Free of Stress,
Inner Conflict, and Self-Sabotage* (McGraw-Hill, 2006)

*The Now Habit: A Strategic Program for Overcoming
Procrastination and Enjoying Guilt-Free Play*
(Tarcher/Penguin, 2007)

Audio CDs

*Conquering Procrastination: How to Stop Stalling
and Start Achieving* (Nightingale-Conant, 2008)

Productivity Engineering and Mental Toughness
(Hypnosisnetwork.com, 2006)

The Now Habit, Unabridged (GildanMedia, 2007)

Coping with the Emotional Impact of Cancer

Become an Active Patient and Take Charge of Your Treatment

Neil A. Fiore, Ph.D.

WITHDRAWN

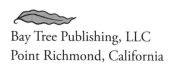
Bay Tree Publishing, LLC
Point Richmond, California

© 1984, 1986, 1990, 2009 by Neil A. Fiore, Ph.D.

Portions of this book appeared under the title, *The Road Back to Health*.

All rights reserved. Printed in the United States of America. No part of this book may be reproduced or transmitted in any form or by any means, electronic or mechanical, including photocopying, recording, or by any information storage and retrieval systems, without written permission from the publisher. For information, contact www.baytreepublish.com

Library of Congress Cataloging-in-Publication Data

Fiore, Neil A.

Coping with the emotional impact of cancer : become an active patient and take charge of your treatment / by Neil A. Fiore.
    p. cm.
Rev. ed. of: Road back to health / Neil A. Fiore. 1990.
Includes bibliographical references and index.

ISBN 978-0-9801758-3-7

1. Cancer--Psychological aspects. I. Fiore, Neil A. Road back to health. II. Title.

RC263.F5268 2009

This book is dedicated to the patients and families who could benefit from holistic medical care that treats not only their illness but also the healthy aspects of their bodies as well as their mind and emotions.

This book is also dedicated to the volunteers and workers in so many programs that now lend support to cancer patients and their families—groups such as The Wellness Community, Make Today Count, I Can Cope, Susan G. Komen for the Cure, the Lance Armstrong Foundation, and to the National Coalition for Cancer Survivorship.

Contents

Foreword
to the First Edition

Whenever the diagnosis is cancer, and perhaps any serious illness, the patient is immediately faced, at this most inopportune of times, with making many decisions which may effect the course of the illness. Although very few cancer patients are aware of it, one significant decision they must make is whether to become a partner with their physician in the fight for recovery or be a hopeless, helpless, passive spectator in this, the most important battle in which they will ever engage. Within The Wellness Community, we call those who choose to be a part of the battle "Patients Active," and those who turn it all over to their health care professionals "Patients Passive."

So that there can be no misunderstanding, it is the basic tenet of The Wellness Community that medical attention is primary and that psychosocial services are secondary and adjunctive. Also, so that there can be no possibility of a judgment being read into those terms, I hasten to say that there is no "good" or "bad," "right" or "wrong" choice. I believe, in the very fiber of my being, that whatever decision the individual makes is perfect for that individual.

However, because of misinformation about cancer which has existed for over 200 years and has become an integral part of our culture, most cancer patients become "Patients Passive" because they have ingrained in them the belief that they have no alternative. They believe they have no choice but to be passive.

As Dr. Fiore illustrates in this most compelling story of his bout with and recovery from cancer, that's just not true. There are many ways cancer patients can act as partners with their health care teams which will, at the very least, improve the quality of their lives and may enhance the possibility of recovery. There's the point! *Dr. Fiore serves humanity and the reader with cancer well by making it very clear, through his own example, that cancer patients, and perhaps all others facing life-threatening illness, (1) can play a most significant* part *in their fight for recovery, and (2) that the part they play may have a beneficial effect* on *the course of the illness, (3) and will improve the quality of their lives; (4) that they have nothing to lose and everything to gain by at least deciding what course to follow instead of blindly assuming that they must be passive; and finally (5) that they are not at fault or to blame. Whatever happens.*

I have read too many books and articles over the past several years which imply or say straight out that the cancer patient is somehow at fault for the onset of the illness, or for the illness not progressing as hoped. There is absolutely no basis, either scientific or anecdotal, for either statement even assuming, as do most modern scientists, that behavior may play a part in the onset or the course of the illness.

To be to blame for the onset of the illness, the patient must have participated in some activity while *knowing* that such activity could result in cancer. He or she must have taken a conscious risk *knowing* that cancer could be the result. Unless we are discussing smoking or overexposure to the sun, I have never met a cancer patient who was aware of taking such a risk.

Neither is the cancer patient at fault if the course of the disease does not progress toward health. Although there is reason to believe that the patient can participate in actions which may enhance the possibility of recovery, no matter what anyone says, there is no behavioral formula a cancer patient can follow which assures recovery. Since there is no "right" way to act, the cancer patient cannot be at fault, because there is no "wrong" or "inadequate" way to act. *But since these positive emotions and activities improve the quality of life, have no unpleasant side effects and may* alter the course of the illness toward health *there is every reason in the world to give them a try.*

Dr. Fiore did just that and tells us about his efforts and their results—without symptoms for over 14 years at this writing—in concise and clear prose. He does all this while staying well within the bounds of accepted medical protocol. Hurrah for this inspiring life and this rational and interesting book about that life.

—Harold H. Benjamin, Ph.D.
Founder, The Wellness Community

Preface

When I was diagnosed with "terminal" cancer on June 13, 1974, my doctors were not prepared to treat the emotional and psychological aspects of my condition. Nor were there books to tell me what to expect, how to cope, and what I could do to improve the quality, if not the length, of my life. In the thirty-five years since I survived that diagnosis and treatment, I have seen major improvements in the holistic treatment of patients and hundreds of helpful books, websites, and articles become available to help patients cope.

There remains, however, the need for a message about coping with the emotional impact of illness that does not blame the patient or cavalierly speculates about how thoughts or emotions might cause disease. *Coping with the Emotional Impact of Cancer* is an attempt to fill that gap. It is based on what I've learned as a patient, but more than that, it includes what I've learned as a psychotherapist working with hundreds of patient diagnosed with serious illness, and from the research literature.

From the beginning of my experience with cancer, I felt that I was fortunate to have training in psychology, self-hypnosis, focusing, and visualization. These equipped me to cope with the emotional and physical impact of this life-threatening illness. I feel an obligation, therefore, to communicate to you what I've learned.

I also feel a responsibility to educate medical caregivers about the patient's perspective and the patient's need for emotional support. Though I was anxious about questioning my doctors, I was able to challenge some of their decisions and to remain an active participant in my healthcare. Because I was unusually equipped to deal with an overwhelming medical diagnosis and procedure, I feel an additional responsibility to speak up for all patients and to inform our caregivers of our needs as patients.

My active participation in my treatment decisions caused my oncologist to ask me to make a videotape to tell other cancer patients how I coped with chemotherapy and its side effects. The script I wrote for that videotape led to recommendations to my doctors and a presentation at hospital grand rounds. Subsequent speeches—entitled "Coping with a Life-Threatening Illness" and "Becoming an Active Patient"—encouraged me to write "Fighting Cancer—One Patient's Perspective," which was published in February 1979, volume 300 edition of *The New England Journal of Medicine.*

In 1982, I was asked to contribute to a research project at the University of California Medical Center in San Francisco for patients afflicted with melanoma. My job was to conduct couples and group counseling for patients and their families to help them cope with the stress of cancer and its treatment. In this book, I have attempted to include you and your family in our sessions on coping with the emotional impact of cancer and other serious illnesses.

—Neil Fiore

How to Use This Book

The Introduction gives you a brief history of how I coped with cancer and demonstrates the power of becoming an active patient.

Chapters 1 and 2—"Coping with Your Diagnosis" and "The Power of Your Beliefs"—will give you tools to understand and manage your initial shock at hearing your diagnosis. You will also be equipped with new ways of thinking about cancer and how robust your body can be in working with medical treatments to beat cancer.

Chapter 3, "Maintaining a Fighting Spirit: What You Can Do," empowers you to take charge of your initial reactions so you can make more energy available for coping and healing. You will learn five actions you can take to lessen your stress and worry by giving attention to the 99 percent of you that is healthy and fighting your illness.

Chapter 4, "Managing the Stress of Serious Illness," provides essential tools that prepare your body for surgery and other treatments by lowering stress hormones. You will also learn how to speak to yourself in a compassionate voice that creates the inner safety needed to lessen your fears and worries.

Chapter 5, "Coping with Depression and Helplessness," explains why these natural feelings follow an overwhelming shock and how you can acknowledge and manage them. While physical illness is not a psychological disease, medication for depression and anxiety are often helpful in keeping you active and involved in your life.

Chapter 6, "Becoming an Active Patient," will encourage you to participate at whatever level you wish in your own healthcare and medical decisions. Your feelings and thoughts are valid considerations in optimizing the outcome of your holistic treatment. Active participation is a powerful medicine in itself in overcoming depression and anxiety.

Chapter 7, "You and Your Doctor," is about building a working relationship with your doctors, nurses, and healthcare workers. What is often missing from this relationship is your input as the patient and your ability to choose and commit to the recommended treatments. To participate more fully in your healthcare you'll need to protect yourself from the misuse of statistics. You may also want to round out your treatment by including professionals who can give you information about nutrition and psychosocial support.

Chapter 8, "Communication Skills," will help you to express your feelings in ways that keep you connected to your healthcare professionals and your family. Learning to speak about difficult topics can be uncomfortable at first but will help you lower stress and maintain contact with others instead of becoming isolated.

Chapter 9, "Fully Alive after Cancer," deals with the process of survival, the fear of recurrence, and how to stay fully alive after being diagnosed with a serious illness.

Today, diseases such as cancer are no longer a death sentence. Most people diagnosed with a life-threatening disease will live with their disease under control for many years. Some will be cured and will return to a healthy life. This chapter will prepare you to face the challenges of making the transition to a new lease on life.

Chapter 10, "Coping with End of Life Issues," presents the challenges that arise in the last stage of life. Though you most likely will live many healthy years beyond your diagnosis, it is often helpful to face the fear of those last days with a plan and the knowledge that any pain can be managed.

Coping with the Emotional Impact of Cancer is designed to provide you and your family with a guide through the emotional and psychological impact of a life-threatening diagnosis and treatment. It offers you new coping mechanisms, perhaps requiring that you leave behind less effective ones. It can also enhance your sense of effectiveness in the world and give greater control over your reactions during a time when both may feel hopelessly out of control.

It is my sincerest hope that you will find this book helpful in coping with the emotional impact of serious, life-threatening illness and that it will provide you with the tools to return more fully alive to the joys of everyday life.

Acknowledgements

I would like to express my gratitude to the doctors, nurses, and hospital staff at Kaiser-Permanente, Oakland , California , whose medical skill and dedication helped save my life. I also am grateful for their support of my active participation in my medical care at the time of my cancer and for more than thirty-five years as a cancer survivor.

The editors of *The New Journal of Medicine* deserve acknowledgment for their willingness to publish my article, "Fighting Cancer: One Patient's Perspective," in 1979 when patient advocacy and the open discussion of the psycho-emotional aspects of cancer treatment were still in their infancy.

I am indebted to the early researchers and authors of seminal works regarding the human side of cancer, most especially, Dr. Jimmie Holland and Ada Rogers, R.N., of Memorial Sloan-Kettering; Dr. Ernest Rosenbaum of San Francisco; Dr. Cicely Saunders of St. Christopher's Hospice, London; Dr. Fran Lewis of the University of Washington, Seattle; and Dr. David Spiegel of Stanford.

I must acknowledge the support of the late Norman Cousins who wrote the foreword and Hal Benjamin who wrote the preface to *The Road Back to Health*, and the late Grace Bechtold of Bantam Books who, over 25 years ago, believed that the public needed a book that speaks to the emotional aspects of cancer.

I also wish to thank my current publisher, David Cole, of Bay Tree Publishing, for encouraging me to write a new, updated version of a book that supports cancer patients and their families through the difficulties and transformative possibilities of facing this life-threatening illness.

Important Note: The identities of the patients and clients mentioned in this book have been altered to protect their confidentiality.

Introduction

How a Psychologist Coped
with His Own Cancer

At the age of thirty-two a doctor told me that I had one year to live. I had a fast-growing cancer that had spread to my left lung. My reactions were probably similar to those of anyone who's been diagnosed with a life-threatening illness, except that I had faced death nine years earlier as a paratrooper with the 101st Airborne in Vietnam. This, when combined with my training as a psychologist, gave me an advantage and additional tools for coping with the stress, worries, and emotional impact of cancer.

My training as a therapist also gave me insight into the perspective and reactions of my doctors and nurses, as well as how my own reactions might help or hinder me in a battle for my life. Over the years, I learned how my own patients' emotions and beliefs affected their ability to cope with their careers, relationships, and medical conditions. I found it difficult to understand, therefore, why so many of the doctors and hospitals seemed to ignore the emotional and psychological aspects of their patients during the diagnosis, treatment, coping, and recovery processes.

While my experiences may seem unusual, I have found in my work with hundreds of patients coping with serious and chronic illnesses that many of these experiences are quite common. Though this introduction focuses primarily on my own experience with cancer and its medical treatment, it is my hope that you will apply its hard-won lessons to any illness or medical situation.

Discovering My Cancer

My journey in coping with cancer began more than three months before I ever saw a doctor. I later discovered that both patients and doctors with cancer symptoms delay seeking treatment, on average, three months after they become aware of the early signs. My only symptom was a discomfort in my groin when I showered or crossed my legs. Otherwise, I felt healthy and kept very active jogging, playing tennis, and skiing. Although I knew something was wrong, I didn't know what kind of doctor to see for a pain "down there" until a friend told me that he was going to see a urologist (a specialist who deals with the urinary or uro-genital tract) for a similar pain.

Finding a Doctor

By the spring of 1974, it became apparent that the lump and pain near my right testicle were not going away and that I should see a doctor. I was hoping that the lump was only an infection that could be treated with an antibiotic.

With my friend's encouragement, I made an appointment to see an urologist. The first doctor I saw treated me as if I were a specimen. Instead of speaking to me as he examined my testicle, called over a resident, pointed out what he called a "calcification" (a hard deposit of calcium salts surrounding irritated tissue), and began talking to him about cancer and surgery. I had come to the hospital for antibiotics for what I thought was simple infection, but, without ever checking with me, this doctor talked to the intern about exploratory surgery and removing my testicle for precautionary reasons. My grandmother had died of cancer. I thought of it as a disease for old people. I was too young to have cancer and was not prepared for the shock of hearing that, this time, I was the one diagnosed with the "Big C."

I was equally shocked and frightened by this doctor's lack of regard for me as his patient. I had read about people who had breasts and limbs removed during what were supposed to be simply biopsies or exploratory surgery. I now could see how patients lose control over the medical decisions and surgery that would affect them for the rest of their lives. In that moment, I resolved to not let that happen to me. As soon as I could get away from this doctor, I went to the head nurse and asked her who else I could see in the Urology Department. I had just fired my first doctor, and I was eager to seek a second opinion and more humane medical treatment.

I was frightened, but not ready to give up control of my life to the doctors. With the heightened vigilance that comes from fighting to survive a life-threatening situation, I carefully watched their behavior and interpreted their motives.

I know that many doctors are very caring, but mine seemed to have the narrow focus of men with a mission. Their dedication to fighting cancer reminded me of the generals I had seen in Vietnam—a little too self-important and willing to risk the lives of others out of their own sense of zeal for a cause. From the way the doctors talked, I got the impression that cancer is something that resides outside the body of a living, feeling human being—something like the fear of Communism in Vietnam that they needed to attack with knives, chemicals, and B-52 strikes.

Whenever I could, I attempted to lessen the doctor's sense that he had complete responsibility for my life. I wanted to demonstrate that I could participate in my own healthcare. I asked questions about the treatment process they were considering and indicated that I would have to think about the consequences of any treatments before consenting to any of them.

Each recommendation they made seemed to involve a lengthening the amount of time I would be in pain and gave me only a slightly greater chance of surviving beyond one year.

The doctors were acting as if I were near death or completely cancerous. But, the strange fact was that I felt pretty good. Though I could accept that about one percent of my body was cancerous, I reasoned that the other 99 percent was healthy. I wondered, "What about the healthy side of me and its ability to fight cancer? Who's going to consider that part of me and rally its support, if not me?"

A Second, and a Third, Opinion

After I fired my first urologist, the head nurse referred me to a doctor who was willing to talk directly to me about my surgery and cancer therapy options. Even then, I insisted on asking him about the procedures and gaining his agreement that the testicle would be removed only if it was cancerous. I appreciated that he talked to me openly and informed me of the possible stages of treatment following exploratory surgery and possible removal of my right testicle. They included:

1. A lymph node dissection—an eight-hour operation in which most of the lymph nodes are removed from the center of the body along with the appendix and spleen

2. Removal of the lower portion of my left lung

3. Chemotherapy and, possibly,

4. Radiation

I asked him dozens of questions about the potential side effects of surgery and chemotherapy, the reasons for each procedure, and the research that indicated that these procedures would improve my odds of beating cancer. That's when my doctor stopped my questioning and shouted, "Surgery is scheduled for tomorrow morning!"

At that moment, I heard a disembodied voice from deep inside me say, "No, doctor, surgery is not scheduled for tomorrow morning. I haven't talked to my family and I haven't gotten a second and a third opinion."

I don't know what kept me from panicking at the thought of all the torturous tests that lay ahead of me. Maybe I was able to stay calm because I knew I was stubborn enough to refuse any treatment that didn't make sense to me. I also knew that I wouldn't allow their fear of death propel me into useless attempts at conquering cancer. Instead, I would consider each phase as it came to me from the new perspective gained with each step. I would focus on the present and on my current condition, not on the imagined "terminal" stage or the need for dozens of tests and painful therapies in the future.

Facing Surgery

Before agreeing to surgery, I consulted with three other oncologists, each of whom advocated for their favorite treatment—surgery, chemotherapy, or radiation. It was hard to know who to believe. I was learning that medical science is more of an art than a science and that doctors truly cannot make god-like, perfect decisions. I would have to rely on myself to make the ultimate decisions.

When X-rays revealed a spot in my left lung, I knew that there was a strong probability that the lump in my groin was malignant and spreading. Now—after considering several expert opinions—I was convinced that exploratory surgery was necessary to determine if the growth was in fact cancerous.

Following a talk with my new urologist, surgery was scheduled. If I had not consulted with other doctors and had not done some reading, I would have felt pressured into having surgery. Luckily, I took time to consider my feelings and asked many questions the prior week. Though this was not what I *wanted* to do, and definitely not my favorite thing to do, I now felt that, given the circumstances, I could freely *choose* surgery.

I called my closest friend and let him know that I was going into the hospital for exploratory surgery for a possible cancerous growth. I notified my supervisor at work and decided that I would not call my family on the East Coast until I had more information. I reasoned that I didn't want to trouble them while they were three thousand miles away and unable to do much except worry. Then I packed some books and the steno pad I had been using for recording questions for the doctors and had my friend drive me to the hospital.

After several hours of waiting in my hospital room, an attendant came to wheel me down to surgery. It was approximately noon on June 13, 1974. Even though I had been sedated, I was very frightened. Two anxious people were having trouble giving me a spinal anesthetic. I sleepily complied with their orders while fighting off thoughts of being paralyzed by these agitated people. They added to my fright by forcibly pulling my head down and shouting, "Bend over some more. I can't find a good spot."

After surgery, the same people were again agitated and yelling at me to try to move my feet after surgery. I was still anesthetized and couldn't feel a thing. I was truly helpless and certain that they had botched their job. In my drugged state, I was extremely frightened by their insensitivity and by my own inability to communicate my fear. Once again, I was shocked at how medieval and inhumane so-called modern medicine and hospitals can be.

Waking Up During Surgery

While the operation was still in progress, I began to sit up to see what was going on. I saw a panorama of startled faces as I asked if the lump attached to my right testicle was cancerous. A resident pushed me down and told me that, indeed, it was cancerous and that the testicle had been removed. On hearing that, I felt a strange sense of relief and let the anesthetic put me back to sleep while the surgical team finished its work.

During my recovery, I wondered about the sense of relief that came from learning that "exploratory" surgery was necessary to confirm that I really had cancer. At the time, I felt that the relief came from knowing that I hadn't submitted to unnecessary surgery and that I hadn't allowed my testicle to be removed for no reason. There was no need, therefore, to blame myself for permitting what could have been an unnecessary mutilation. I thought, "What an incredible tyrant I must be with myself if I feel relieved at not incurring my own anger!"

A Return of Meaning to Life

Later, I realized that some of the relief came from my belief that the doctor had removed the cancer at an early stage. And, part came from discovering that, in spite of feeling damaged by cancer and surgery, I really wanted to live to help others cope with similar experiences. A sense of meaning and urgency about life had returned. When I was going through some very stressful times at work and in my relationships, my life had lost some of its joy and purpose. But, when faced with the likelihood of death, I was ecstatic to discover that I was overwhelmingly in favor of life, and a life that refused to submit to a passive patient role and to the usual hospital treatment.

Following surgery, I underwent a series of tests to see how far the cancer had spread and to determine if I were strong enough to withstand chemotherapy, radiation, and additional surgery.

One of these tests was to determine if cancer had spread through the lymphatic system to the brain. It involved the removal of a lymph node from each side of my neck under local anesthetic. Because of the way the doctor carried out the surgery, it was one of the most gruesome procedures I experienced. The surgeon in charge was teaching a resident how to locate the nodes with his fingers. I was conscious while these two people fished in both sides of my neck with an array of clamps and instruments that felt as if someone had emptied a tool chest of wrenches and screwdrivers into an open wound. It took them much longer than usual to locate the nodes, but the surgeon assured the resident that she never gives up.

I was perspiring heavily and was soaking wet. My stomach and neck muscles were strained from the position I had to hold. I thought I was going to lose my mind. I kept trying to concentrate on something pleasant as I had taught myself in self-hypnosis and meditation. But, the surgeon kept bringing my attention back to what she was doing, and kept telling me, "Meditation and hypnosis don't work."

I had assumed incorrectly that because the surgeon was a woman she would be more sensitive to the feelings of her patients. I was angry at her for being another insensitive doctor and at myself for letting my guard down and having different expectations of a female surgeon.

Different Agendas

While recuperating from surgery and from the tests, I wrote down questions I wanted to ask my doctor. If I didn't write things down, I would be too shocked by his latest announcement or too timid in the face of his apparent busyness to remember the question or the answer. He answered most of my questions and gave me the research references upon which he was basing his treatment plan for me. As soon as I was released from the hospital, I went to the medical library and looked up anything I could find about my type of cancer, an embryonal carcinoma. I realized that I could trust my doctor to be acquainted with the latest research and the least damaging procedures.

I learned from him and from my reading that a lymph node dissection could hit certain nerves, resulting in an inability to ejaculate. In addition, radiation and chemotherapy could cause sterility. Being still new to how hospitals and doctors view what is important for the patient, I was shocked to learn that they didn't take the issue of sterility seriously and were not informed about sperm banks at that time.

It was becoming increasingly clear to me that we had different agendas and goals. I was intending to live a long life, with minimal damage to the quality of that life from cancer treatment, and I wanted the option of having children. They, however, were willing to do anything to me I would allow and could withstand, in order to ensure that they had killed the cancer. The side effects and lasting effects of the surgery and treatments were not their concern. If I survived five years, regardless of how, they had done their job. Now, my sense of purpose was even more emboldened. For the sake of myself and future patients, I had to convince my doctors to consider the emotional impact of cancer and cancer therapies.

Fighting to Get Chemotherapy

Recovery from surgery went well, and now it was time to decide which therapies were needed to eliminate whatever cancer cells may have spread to other regions of my body.

My surgeon told me that the next step would be the removal of my lymph nodes in an eight-hour operation that would cause much discomfort and would delay my ability to start chemotherapy. He said that the research indicated that this procedure would raise my odds of survival from ten percent to thirty percent.

From my reading about treating testicular cancers, I was prepared to argue against the lymph node operation unless my doctor could convince me that this procedure would substantially increase my chances of survival.

As it turned out, my lymph nodes appeared cancer-free on both a lymph angiogram (a diagnostic test in which a dye is injected into the lymphatic channels to make the nodes visible on an X-ray) and in the pathologist's analysis of the two nodes removed from my neck. An additional X-ray, however, revealed that a second spot showed up on my left lung within two weeks. This was an almost certain sign, I believed, that the cancer was rapidly spreading through my bloodstream where it was being filtered and held by the lungs.

When I arrived for my post-surgery appointment, I discovered that the chief surgeon was filling in for my doctor who was on vacation. He encouraged me to go through with the lymph node surgery and suggested that we wait to see if more spots appeared in the lung. After all, he reasoned, the lung could be surgically removed.

Surgeons want to do surgery, I reminded myself, and radiation therapists want to do radiation. As the psychologist Abraham Maslow said, "If the only tool you have is a hammer, you tend to treat every problem as if it's a nail."

Luckily, I had done my homework. I argued that cancer was not spreading through my lymph nodes. The spots in my lungs were evidence that they were doing their job of filtering the blood stream and holding onto cancer cells, just as the lymphatic system holds onto any debris coming its way. I needed a treatment that cleared my blood stream of cancer, not lymph node surgery that would delay the start of chemotherapy and leave me with more spots on my lungs. Chemotherapy should begin immediately in order to stop the spread of cancer through my blood stream.

It was this positive belief in my body that contributed to a medical decision that saved my life.

Much to my surprise, the chief surgeon quickly agreed that what I said made sense. At which point I pounded my fist on his desk and told him, "I want to start chemotherapy today!" He then made the necessary arrangements to put me on what was then an experimental chemotherapy protocol. I was frightened about the second spot on my lung but was relieved to be spared a complicated eight-hour lymph node operation and to enter the long fight with most of my lymphatic system intact.

Chemotherapy Begins

Having made my point with the surgeon, and being all too aware that there was now a second spot on my lung, I was eager to begin chemotherapy immediately. I called the oncology-chemotherapy department to see when I could take the tests that would determine if my body could withstand drugs that were experimental and "toxic." They told me that I should call back after the Fourth of July holiday. Somehow, the calm voice of the receptionist lulled me into believing that my condition wasn't serious and that I could wait a few more days.

As luck would have it, I had scheduled one more second opinion with another oncologist. When I told him of my case and the delay of chemotherapy, he shouted with great passion in a Persian accent,

"You're a cancer patient. There are no holidays for you!" His strong reaction and his very welcomed expression of emotion woke me up to the fact that I must not allow myself to be seduced into a casual attitude about fighting for my life.

Immediately after our appointment, I called the chemotherapy department and told them, "I'm a cancer patient and can't wait until after July Fourth to start chemotherapy." We met that day and scheduled my first injection. Within three weeks of surgery I was taking my first treatment of very powerful drug-cocktail of Adriamycin, Velban, and Bleomycin.

Each week for eight months I went to the hospital for a blood test and an injection. Each week the veins in my arm became narrower and more scarred by the corrosive drugs. Each week finding a vein for the blood test and for the injection became increasingly difficult. Each week became a little hell of pain, fear, self-recrimination for cowardice, lack of understanding from the medical staff, and alienation.

Yet, it was all worth it because after the second injection, the spots on my lung were no longer visible on the X-ray. I was ecstatic. I felt triumphant. But these feelings were short-lived. The irony is that the drugs were so effective that I now found it more difficult to complete the series of injections because there was no visible evidence of cancer cells in my body. I was told that I needed to complete the entire eight-month protocol of planned injections in order to mop up any "microscopic foci" that remained in my body. No one could be sure when I would be completely clean or how much risk was involved in stopping the treatment early. Though I felt optimistic that most of the cancer cells had been removed, thereby reducing the "tumor load" my healthy body had to deal with, I chose to stay on the experimental drugs. I made this decision because of the danger that the cancer could return if I prematurely ended chemotherapy and out of a sense of duty to future cancer patients who might benefit from the research.

My doctor and nurse told me that the drugs were highly toxic and that the side effects included nausea, loss of hair, blisters on the tongue, vomiting, and fever and chills. However, I didn't experience the usual side effects until after the fifth or sixth injection. Remember, I had argued with the chief surgeon to put me on chemotherapy. I wasn't repeating to myself, "I have to take chemotherapy. They're making me do this." I fought to get it, I chose it, and I asked that it start immediately. My attitude lessened any inner conflict, ambivalence, and stress that comes from telling yourself, "You have to do something you don't want to do."

No doubt, my active participation in my treatment lowered my stress hormones and improved my body's ability to cope. In addition, I was in good physical condition and hoped that I could endure the treatments with limited side effects. The chemotherapy staff, however, repeatedly told me that I, too, would soon lose my hair and become nauseous, just like every other person who takes chemo.

I couldn't understand why they were so afraid of my optimism. They seemed overzealous in carrying out their duty of warning patients of possible side effects. They made it sound predetermined, and as if having hope was naive.

As I look back on how they reacted to me, I wonder if they felt a need to protect themselves from being too hopeful about their patients. Thirty years ago, over fifty percent of their patients were dying of cancer. Is it any wonder that they would fear being too optimistic even today when over sixty-five percent survive and live with cancer?

They're afraid of giving false hope and, therefore, often err in the direction of dire predictions that are repeatedly proven wrong by so-called "terminal" cases like mine. In an attempt to stop my doctor's negative predictions, I told him that I promised I wouldn't haunt him if I died of cancer after he gave me hope that I might survive it.

The Long Fight

With the start of chemotherapy, my involvement in decision-making and choice of treatments seemed to end. I became passive. Even the power I felt from living each moment began to diminish as it became apparent that I would live if I could withstand the treatment. Soon, I slipped back into worrying about the future and about what others thought of me.

I was no longer choosing chemotherapy. It became something I made myself do. Each week I would sadly drag myself to the hospital for my injection, hope that the nurse would quickly find a vein, and try not to get nauseous at the first smell of the alcohol swab used to clean the injection site. I would try to relax, hoping that that would keep my veins from constricting. I would exhale hard and try not to think about how toxic the chemicals were and of the damage they were doing to my veins and internal organs.

When my hair began to fall out in clumps, and when each injection of chemotherapy was followed by vomiting most of the night, I started to feel depressed and helpless. Not only wasn't I choosing my treatment, I had lost control of how long it was going to last. Miscalculations of how much medication I was supposed to receive led to disappointment after deep disappointment, as the number of shots were continually increased.

I had made a chart with a blank thermometer that I would fill in by degrees, each gradation representing the completion of a chemotherapy shot. Each week I looked forward to coloring in another shot on the thermometer with a red pen. But when the doctor started increasing the total number of shots, I could no longer bear making the corrections. I cried, tore it up, and threw it out.

He then told me about how we were going to make sure we licked this cancer and that chemotherapy would be followed with radiation and the lymph node operation that I thought I had escaped. I had felt so proud of how I handled the initial stages of my cancer, and now it felt totally out of my control. This was a real low point for me, physically and emotionally. I took out my frustration and anger on a punching bag I hung in my garage. I started to hit the bag with a series of one-two punches and then reminded myself that this fight would take more than a simple one-two punch. It required that I train myself to keep punching until I was completely exhausted.

In mid-September of 1974, after two and a half months of chemotherapy, I entered the hospital with a fever of unknown origin and remained there for ten days while tests were performed to determine the cause of my 104-degree fever. I felt and looked like a mess. The chemotherapy had caused my hair and beard to fall out in clumps. It was so depressing to wake up with new patches of hair on my pillow that I decided to shave my head and face completely clean. I was getting very little sleep because profuse sweating required me to change the sheets and my clothing several times during the night. I was very weak and frightened. This was the sickest I'd ever been, and I didn't know if the fever was caused by advancing cancer. (We now know that a fever can marshal the immune system's white cells to fight infection and inflammation.)

I desperately fought my sense of helplessness by doing whatever I could. I took my own temperature every waking hour and recorded it to become familiar with its fluctuations. After taking a series of medical tests that were administered without any sensitivity to my need for rest, I announced that I would need to know the reason for each additional test before I would agree to it. I refused to go to the X-ray department at a time when my temperature was at its peak, knowing that I would have to wait in a drafty hall while my clothes and sheets would be soaked wet with sweat.

My need for some sense of control and dignity became so crucial that I even refused to have my temperature taken with a rectal thermometer. Remember, I was taking my own temperature orally every hour, and the rationale they offered for preferring the rectal thermometer was that drinking liquids would give an inaccurate reading. I assured them that I could take my own temperature without drinking hot or cold liquids, and that I would no longer consent to any further insults to my body.

I'm sure they thought that I was being an awful nuisance. But it seemed quite clear to me that I was the only one who was going to take proper care of my body and let it have some rest. My body and I were quickly becoming a supportive team. When a nurse said that my refusal to take any additional tests or to be X-rayed on their schedule was irresponsible, I just quietly wept. I was so exhausted I couldn't tell who made sense and who was doing the right thing.

I was becoming more certain, however, that I had to trust my own body more than the medical profession's obsession with tests to ensure that they don't miss a rare disease. I had been subjected to a whole series of tests, and all the results were negative (that is, no disease was found). It was my belief that the fever had to run its course and that if they got a positive test result they would be pleased with themselves, but would only tell me to rest and take liquids. They never did find out what caused the fever, which eventually subsided with no medication other than Tylenol. I'm sure part of my recovery was due to the fact that my body got some rest from the stress of being subjected to additional tests and interrupted sleep.

A Turning Point

While I was trying to recuperate from the fever, I felt a resurgence of the power I had felt when I was actively involved in making decisions about my cancer therapy. Once again, I was reminded that hospitals and bodies have different agendas and different schedules. I was determined to fight for my body and felt physically stronger as I took control over my treatment. This made me wonder if my fever were psychosomatic in origin. Mentally and physically, I needed a rest from chemotherapy. The fever kept me off chemotherapy for three weeks. I decided that if I ever wanted a rest from the drugs again, I would actively state my wishes. It was obvious that I had slipped into thinking that I had to take the drugs for my doctor, and that I was no longer choosing to take them.

I also realized that the repetition of the word toxic to describe my powerful medicines, had naturally made me ambivalent about taking them. I had been placed in a double bind: I was told that the drugs were poisonous and that I had to take this poison to save my life—ignoring the reactions of my stomach, hair, and veins. I decided that if I were going to take these powerful drugs, it would have to be because I chose to, and because I believed they were positive and powerful allies of my body's fight against cancer.

The words of a nutritionist came to mind. He told me, "The reason anticancer drugs cause blisters and hair loss is that they kill rapidly dividing cells. Cancer cells are usually rapidly reproducing, as are the cells of the mucous lining, hair, and skin." From that point on I used the side effects of the drugs as reminders of the power of my allies in the fight against cancer. My healthy hair and skin cells would recover from chemotherapy, but the confused cancer cells would stop reproducing and die.

In addition to deciding that I needed to be in control of whatever medication or test I would take, I also decided that I needed some control over the length of my chemotherapy. Although I had requested a Tumor Board Review—a review of a case by a panel of medical experts from several fields—my doctor didn't follow through. Now I was determined to have a board review my case to support or refute his contention that more chemotherapy was needed along with radiation and the lymph-node dissection. I had to be very persistent, but finally he agreed to set a date for a tumor board review and to hear their recommendations regarding further treatment.

Before he agreed to the review, my oncologist argued that he was responsible for my life and that I didn't have to worry about such decisions. With quite a bit of emotion he proclaimed, "I know a physician with cancer who tried to make his own decisions, and he had a psychotic break." I told him, "I thrive on decisions. And if anything would drive me crazy it would be giving up responsibility for my life!"

I told my doctor that, while I considered him to be an expert in his field, I was the one who would live or die with the consequences of further treatment. I said, "I will have to maintain responsibility for my life, and I will have to make the ultimate decisions."

That intense exchange with my doctor was a turning point in our relationship. Somehow, he seemed less worried about me and more open about his own life and feelings. Eventually, he asked me to make a videotape for other cancer patients, describing how I coped with cancer, cancer treatment, and my own feelings. The film was well received by the patients and the staff, and six months later, I was invited to speak to the doctors at hospital Grand Rounds. Since the recording of that first video, my oncologist has been instrumental in establishing a counseling and patient education program that includes videotapes made by patients with other types of cancers.

The Road Back to Health

The rest of the story moves quickly, with few crises. The tumor board approved of my progress and felt that neither radiation nor the lymph-node dissection would be necessary. It recommended completion of the weekly experimental drugs followed by "maintenance" drugs every six weeks.

In February 1975, eight months after beginning chemotherapy, I started on this program of maintenance injections. Having six weeks between treatments allowed my body to recuperate, and I was able to return to jogging and going to the gym. After each treatment, however, I would feel fatigued and depressed for a week or two. When I was receiving drugs every week, I didn't realize how depressed they made me feel, but at six-week intervals the change was quite dramatic—like having a flu every month.

After ten months of the maintenance drugs, I had a talk with my doctor. These had been months of returning energy and strength followed by periods of lost progress, fatigue, and frustration. I told my doctor that unless he could convince me that drugs, administered at such long intervals, could do more for me than my own unhindered body and psyche, I was ending chemotherapy. The researchers told my doctor that given that I had survived a year and a half with my type of cancer, there was now a ninety-percent chance that I was cured. This prognosis was just the opposite of the 10-percent chance I was given initially. They recommended that I stay on the drugs for another six months to make sure they had killed any remaining cancer cells.

I remembered the goal-thermometer that I had not been able to complete and all the times I had to tell my body, "Hang in there a little while longer." I had made an important contract with my body that I had reneged on four times, each time agreeing with my oncologist to prolong chemotherapy. This time I was determined to keep my promise to my body.

Then, I made and took responsibility for the very difficult decision to end chemotherapy. In no way would I recommend that patients take themselves off radiation or chemotherapy without a thorough consultation and a lot of serious thought. Remember, I had no visible signs of cancer for eighteen months—no signs on X-rays and none in the lymph nodes. In my case, the evidence suggested that the spread of cancer had been halted by an aggressive regimen of chemotherapeutic agents and that I was free of cancer and, possibly, cured.

Meeting with the "What If" Voices

The night before I was to talk with my doctor about stopping chemo, I sat down in my living room with a pad and a pencil and invited all parts of me to participate in helping me make this monumental decision. I especially wanted to hear from all the "what if" voices in my head, the ones that say, "But what if it comes back. What if your doctor and family tell you 'You should have taken more chemo.'"

All of those "what if" voices had to be answered before every part of me would stand behind my final decision—a decision I could live with. While I sat in my living room, it felt as if I was convening a committee of all my inner voices. I closed my eyes and told every part of me that I was about to end chemotherapy unless the doctor could convince me to continue. I had considered the risks of stopping chemotherapy, and I knew I couldn't stop treatment just because some part of me didn't want the pain and disruption chemotherapy caused in my life. But I also knew I couldn't continue taking it just because some part of me was afraid of making a mistake by not following orders. Regardless of which direction I chose, I knew every part of me would have to be committed to the mission.

On my pad, I wrote down what came to me about every possible worry, risk, benefit, and criticism I would face if my decision to stop chemotherapy proved to be a mistake to my family, my doctor, and myself. I imagined each scenario and acknowledged each "What if the cancer comes back?" Most frequently, I responded with, "Yes, that would be awful. Yes, that would really hurt. Yes, I'd probably cry and be upset. And, yet, I won't let it last for long. I'm taking full responsibility for this decision. I can live with the consequences. I won't make myself feel bad."

That night, I reached a new level of integration; every part of me had been heard and now I had a complete team behind my decision to stop chemotherapy. Even the tyrant voice was cooperating. Chemotherapy had saved my life. But, now it was time to give my body a chance on its own.

Lessons Learned—Lessons to Share

In addition to discovering how essential it is to maintain the ability to choose at least some aspects of one's healthcare, cancer taught me a greater respect for my body and my life. I learned that as much as I wanted the doctor to be like a god that could take responsibility for my life, I am the one who will live with the consequences of medical treatment, and, therefore, I must take responsibility for my own life.

My experience with cancer has brought home to me the fact that I am human and that my time is limited—I will die. Having had cancer has better prepared me for both death and for living the rest of my life more fully alive.

It is my sincere wish that you will find this book helpful for yourself and your family in coping with the emotional impact of cancer and other serious illnesses. I hope you will use the lessons I learned to improve both the quality and quantity of your life.

Postscript

In preparing to write this book, I dug through notes from thirty years ago and came across a letter from my oncologist introducing me to the Cancer Tumor Board at the University of California, San Francisco, Medical Center. It stated that I was on experimental chemotherapy protocol 145, that included Adriamycin, Bleomycin, and Velban, administered by injection every week for eight months.

I was one of eight men out of ten on the West Coast who survived on this new chemo-cocktail that yielded an unprecedented survival rate for testicular cancer. This was a massive improvement over the 10 to 30 percent survival rate obtained with surgery without any chemotherapy. Since the late 1970s, chemotherapy has become the treatment of choice for testicular cancer and has led to 90 percent survival on the newer protocols that followed.

Those of us who volunteered for the experimental protocol can feel some satisfaction in knowing that, not only did this difficult weekly treatment cure us of cancer, it led to the chemotherapy that saved Lance Armstrong. While we can't take credit for Lance's Tour de France victories, we are part of the team that proved that at least some very aggressive cancers can be cured. (Lance Armstrong's cancer had spread to his brain and lungs and yet his chemotherapy resulted in a complete cure.)

If you are struggling through chemo today, you might take some comfort in knowing that your commitment to a protocol may help save the life of a future patient with even more advanced cancer. During your most difficult days of cancer treatment this thought may give a sense of meaning to what you're going through.

Chapter 1

Coping with Your Diagnosis

. . . seeing illness as an occasion to make positive changes in your life beyond the disease itself is a creative adaptation to a major life threat. . . . Your illness is an occasion to reevaluate life—a wake-up call, not a death knell. When your life is threatened, take hold and make the most of it; don't give up on it.
—David Spiegel, M.D., *Living Beyond Limits*

The Initial Shock

In the last forty years, cancer survival rates have risen from less than 45 percent to over 65 percent. There is life after the initial shock of a cancer diagnosis! In the twenty-first century, most patients diagnosed with cancer will live free of cancer or with cancer held in remission for years and even decades.

While many diseases and injuries are more severe, traumatic, and fatal than cancer, the stigma we attach to this disease makes the diagnosis of cancer disproportionately terrifying for most. In literature and in common speech, cancer is frequently referred to as something that is out-of-control, insidious, contagious, deadly, spreading, ugly, isolating, or painful. With such associations deeply embedded in our minds, it is only natural that hearing the diagnosis of cancer elicits such strong feelings of dread and anxiety.

The late Rose Bird, Chief Justice of California, wrote of her feelings about her breast cancer diagnosis in 1976:

It is almost impossible to put into words the shock and terror you feel when you learn you have this dreaded disease. Your emotions run the gamut from disbelief to fear to feelings of great loss. Disbelief, because cancer is always something that happens to the next person, not to you. Fear, because everyone living in this society has been conditioned to believe that a diagnosis of cancer is equivalent to a death warrant. It is not true, but that is the popular conception. Accepting our own mortality is difficult under any circumstances. But in a society which finds euphemisms for the very word death, and which encourages its people to pursue youth with a vengeance, it is doubly difficult. We come to the task ill-equipped, and our society does little to help prepare us.

It will take some time before the recent advances made in the detection, treatment, and cure of cancer and in the care of terminal patients begin to erode the attitudes and beliefs that have existed for centuries. In the meanwhile, with the help of our doctors, nurses, and families, we can begin to consider the diagnosis of cancer as meaningless without answers to specific questions, such as: What type of cancer? At what stage? And, what treatments are available?

That is to say, the diagnosis of cancer itself is no longer a certain death sentence. We all need to be reminded of certain facts about cancer today.

- Many types of cancer are curable.

- Many can be contained.

- We can live with many types of cancer for years and even decades.

- Relief from physical pain is almost always possible, even for advanced and terminal cancer.

Deciding to See a Doctor

While we usually think that the worry and stress about cancer begins with the diagnosis, it's important for families and health professionals to realize that for most patients the stress begins much
earlier; that is, with the first suspicions of having cancer. In fact,
patients in an American Cancer Society survey stated that the time
before the diagnosis was the third most stressful time for them. A
possible explanation for this was given by the patients themselves in
their interviews. Some suspected that they had cancer, but still tried
to deal with their early symptoms alone. Others worked so hard
at repressing their feelings and worries about their symptoms that
they felt they had nothing to talk about.

Even before you decide to see a doctor, you probably worried that
something was wrong—a growth, a spot, or an uncomfortable sen-
sation. With all the information about the warning signs of cancer
that is available in magazines and on the Internet, TV and the radio,
it is almost impossible not to worry about having cancer if you have
any of the symptoms. Yet the average lag-time between first noticing a cancer symptom and seeking a medical consultation is three
months. This is true for laymen and physicians alike, which suggests that medical knowledge of the symptoms and consequences
of cancer isn't necessarily enough to motivate a patient to seek immediate help.

Patients delay in seeing a physician for a number of reasons, most
having to do with fear of treatment and lack of faith in the possibility of a cure or improvement. Too often patients are made to feel
guilty for "delaying," and then they worry about having endangered
their lives. Blame and recrimination implied by the word *delay* are
hardly beneficial. An alternative term, *lag-time*, implies that psychological, emotional, and cognitive adjustments are taking place
during this time, and that many experience stress and worry even
before a clear diagnosis is received.

Certainly, early treatment ought to be sought for any symptom associated with a serious illness, but since the growth and spread of cancer varies considerably, there is no clear evidence that specific time lapses worsen the prognosis of all forms of cancer.' Most patients see a doctor within three months after noticing an abnormality, but a lag-time of more than that may not mean that patients are significantly endangering their lives.

However, for those cancers that are relatively curable at an early stage—colon, breast, some forms of melanoma, and carcinoma of the cervix and uterus—a delay may make a difference in the severity of the disease, its treatment, and in the chance of survival. For other sites—the lungs, pancreas, prostate, esophagus, stomach, and brain—a delay of diagnosis and treatment may be less significant.

Even if you are aware of a cancer symptom, you cannot diagnose on your own the type of cancer, its stage, or know what treatments are available. With cancer, and any serious illness, irrespective of type, "the earlier the better" is the attitude that should be taken about seeking a medical examination.

Greater efforts are needed on the part of medical associations, hospitals, and public health educators to inform the public of preventative health care and cancer-screening techniques such as breast self-exams, testicle self-exams, and occult blood tests for signs of cancer of the colon and rectum.

From my experience in counseling dozens of patients who have delayed in seeking medical advice, even after they were aware of cancer symptoms, I believe that the public needs more than just education about the warning signs.

People need to know how to cope with

- their fear of having cancer;

- their fear of cancer treatment; and,

- their fear of losing control to the doctor and the hospital.

As doctors begin to encourage patients to play a more active role in their healthcare decisions, perhaps we'll find that patients will seek medical advice earlier, when their odds of survival are greater.

When hospitals and doctors offer patient-centered care, we can expect a decrease in patient fears, a lessening of feelings of helplessness, and, possibly, an increase in immune system strength.

Preparing to See a Doctor

If you find yourself procrastinating about seeing a doctor about a potential cancer symptom, you may benefit from an examination of the fears that are keeping you from acting. As in the following example of one woman's experience, you may need to become aware of your initial reactions and prepare yourself for a potential cancer diagnosis.

A friend casually told me that she had a suspicious Pap smear and that she was due to find out the results of follow-up tests. "I'm certain everything will be okay," she said. I told her that the odds were strongly in her favor, but something in her tone made me feel that she was not preparing herself for bad news. Her attempt at remaining positive was leaving her wide open for an unsettling shock if the news was bad. She had no idea how she would handle it or what she would do. I cautioned her about two extreme reactions. One would be an alarmist reaction, either from herself or from her doctors, imagining the worst and jumping into an immediate decision, losing sight of the steps that could be taken to make informed decisions. The other extreme would be a denial of the seriousness of the situation and a refusal to do further testing.

My friend had told herself repeatedly that everything would be all right, that cancer couldn't happen to her. When the results indicated evidence of cancer, therefore, she could not accept it as a fact and she didn't think or talk about it for weeks. All along, she had tried to deny what she knew to be true. All alone, she worried about what could happen to her in cancer therapy.

When she was on a vacation and could no longer occupy her mind with her busy schedule at work, it came to her that "this time it *is* me" and "something needs to be done." When she finally faced it, a flood of feelings and emotions were released. She cried for days and couldn't stop shaking. After suffering through an agonizing time of keeping it to herself, she finally told her friends and family, and scheduled her exploratory surgery. She had a small cancerous growth removed, and today she is fine.

Getting the proper care usually involves several steps. Don't overwhelm yourself by trying to do everything at once. You may need to confront your fears and formulate plans. Consider the following points when deciding to see a doctor about a cancer symptom. Each case is different, so any advice given must be general, and you need to consider your own health needs as you read this list.

1. Promise yourself that you will not be pressured into doing anything that doesn't make sense to you. When making decisions that could affect your life, you have every right to seek second and third opinions. Moreover, you can take a few more days to consider alternatives and to adjust emotionally to your new situation.

2. Promise yourself that you will consider the information from your doctor, your friends, and consultants, but that you will decide what steps to take and when to take them. This commitment to yourself will reduce your stress and can greatly improve your confidence in the treatment plan you and your doctor choose. Know that you will not be rushed into anything, nor will you delay.

3. Commit to facing your fears—even when some part of you doesn't want to—and taking the proper action. Delaying will only prolong your stress and may increase your risk. Though you can delegate many of the medical decisions, remind yourself that only you can take responsibility for your life—you cannot delegate that to anyone.

4. Change doctors if you wish. If you find yourself upset or displeased with the way your doctor is treating you, let him or her know. Before incurring the expense of seeking a new

doctor, you may want to give your current doctor the benefit of the doubt and explain why you are displeased. Your doctors are there to serve you and to take care of your health needs. If they refuse to listen, you have the right to fire them. Many sensitive, competent doctors are willing to listen to your questions and to your concerns, even when they are busy and rushed.

Seek the support of your family, a counselor, or a medical social worker for help in gaining a sense of control over your life and over medical decisions. This will make it easier for you to seek medical advice sooner, knowing that whatever you decide to do will be done at your rate, and with consideration of your needs.

Do You Want to Know the Diagnosis?

Doctors and family members may try to protect you from learning about your diagnosis. Most patients, however, know or discover the diagnosis, and when they haven't been told directly, they lose the benefit of communicating their fears and of having any misconceptions corrected. Thus it seems futile to try to keep the truth from most patients. Most will find out, will lose their ability to trust their doctor, and will have to bear their concerns in silence and isolation.

A poignant example of this comes from a young woman with advanced ovarian cancer who for eight months bore the knowledge of her terminal condition in spite of efforts by her doctors and husband to "save her from knowing." As her condition worsened, she worried about her children seeing her dying and eventually shared her fears with her physician. "I haven't been able to discuss it with my husband," she said, "and I'm afraid that it will be very hard for him when he realizes that I have been carrying this alone all this time." Her physician was the late Dr. Cicely Saunders, founder of St. Christopher's Hospice in London, who reassured her, "Love doesn't need words. I think you will find that you have really been sharing it together, and you will just find yourself talking about it one day." The very next day, to the relief of both, the patient and her husband talked openly. They had nine days to share their feelings with no pretense, and then she died with her family around her.

There are no rules on how to handle such an individual and delicate issue. Each person must find his or her own time and way to communicate to loved ones. But, silence will not convey your good intentions, nor will it conceal the truth. As Dr. Saunders reminds us, "The truth from which the patient is 'protected' is the truth with which he is being forced to live in isolation."

Generally, patients have greater strength and knowledge than we give them credit for. For example, when a group was formed in Los Angeles to help the families of cancer patients cope with their emotional stress, patients were not invited. During the first seven months of the group, patients were excluded because the family members and therapists felt that patients would be too threatened and emotionally overwhelmed. They were surprised, however, at what happened when patients were included.

Attendance increased markedly. The reality of the group experience was the opposite of what the therapy team and physicians had imagined and feared. The cancer patients were significantly more open about issues than other family members and felt supported and reassured by the group rather than threatened or overwhelmed. In retrospect, this is an excellent example of how not only family fears, but also health-care professionals' fears can be easily projected onto the cancer patient.

While policies differ from hospital to hospital and from culture to culture, a number of factors contribute to more honest communication from doctors about the diagnosis of cancer. Greater optimism for the survival of cancer patients, greater public knowledge about cancer and its treatment, increased pressure for patient rights, and changes in the doctor-patient relationship have led to a remarkable turnaround in the percentages of doctors who are in favor of telling patients their diagnoses. A questionnaire administered in 1961 found that doctors in a ratio of only one to nine favored telling patients their diagnosis of cancer. Studies in 2005 and 2006 of medical students, doctors, and patients with cancer found 97 percent favored telling or receiving the diagnosis of cancer—a complete reversal of attitude over the last forty years. A survey by the *Journal of Medical Ethics* (2002) found that 100 percent of 127 medical students answering an anonymous questionnaire and 96 percent of law students favored giving information about the diagnosis of cancer if the patient requests it.

How the Diagnosis Is Conveyed

Cancer means different things to different people. For the doctor who deals with cancer every day, it means something very different than it does to the patient who is hearing the diagnosis for the first time.

The question is not whether the truth should be told, but what exactly is the truth? Telling the diagnosis of cancer to a patient who believes that having cancer automatically means death will not communicate the truth if he has a type of cancer that can be treated and probably cured.

In order to have an accurate understanding of your condition and the treatments available, you may need to ask your doctor to tell you the diagnosis in layman's terms. Also, tell your doctor if you don't want to hear a negative prognosis or side effects. The diagnosis should include a statement of the type of cancer, its stage, and the treatments available. This explanation needs to be in language you can understand.

Know the Difference between the Diagnosis and the Prognosis

The prognosis is the doctor's prediction of the patient's prospect for cure, remission, or the amount of time remaining. It too often is delivered along with the diagnosis, which is the classification of the patient's disease (that is, the type of cancer cell and its stage of growth). Part of the diagnosis should include the treatment plan, which will tell you what tests and treatments to expect.

A treatment plan or the "staging of treatments" makes it clear that something can be done for you and that the odds of your survival and cure can be more accurately determined after each treatment step over the course of weeks or months.

Remind your doctor that statistics are based on old research that includes a group of dozens, hundreds, or thousands of patients who may have had a worse condition than yours with fewer medical tools than are available today. Statistics apply to a group but may not fit you, your current condition, and your advanced medical options.

When patients say they're concerned about their odds, I often tell them, "Regardless of the odds, your job is to do the best you can to improve your odds." Even when patients ask about their chances of survival, as I did myself, I feel that they are asking:

- What can I do to help improve my odds?

- Should I just prepare to die, or should I fight?

- Will this treatment improve my odds and outweigh the risks and suffering?

- Is there any hope for medical advances in the next year or two that could put this disease into remission?

One patient, who outlived her prognosis by many years, has words of warning about doctors' predictions.

> I would also be very cautious when someone tells you how long you have to live. No one knows how long anyone is going to live at any given time. It's a mistake for someone to tell you that you have a certain number of months or years to live because no one can really know that. I'm speaking from experience on that point. I was given one year to live. Well, that was seven

years ago and I'm still here. When a doctor puts a time limit on someone's life, he must realize he's not God. At the end of the year, when I was supposed to die and I was still alive, it was very hard to cope. It was nice, but still very hard. Between the initial diagnosis and death, there's a lot of living to do. If people could just accept this fact, it would make it a lot easier for us cancer patients.

Coping with the Impact of the Diagnosis

The impact of the cancer diagnosis is often experienced as something similar to a physical assault. Recalling their initial reactions, patients have told me:

- When I heard the word *cancer,* it was like a slap in the face.

- It knocked the wind out of me.

- I went into a daze and didn't hear anything else the doctor said.

The numbing effect of the shock of the diagnosis seems to serve the function of temporarily insulating these patients, giving them an opportunity to adjust to what would be a major life change.

Accompanying the shock is often a surprise that being labeled a cancer patient doesn't immediately kill you. In fact, it doesn't necessarily make you feel sick! It is quite possible to feel healthy when you're diagnosed with cancer.

Following the initial shock or surprise, most patients gradually, and at their own pace, come to the realization that some important things may be done in order to cope with this new label of cancer patient. The work of the initial phase of coping with cancer, for both patients and their families, involves making medical decisions, coping with fears and almost unbearable feelings, and caring for each other. Patients and their families benefit enormously by accepting as normal a wide range of feelings, fears, and reactions that accompany the initial shock of the cancer diagnosis, and by openly communicating about them.

I had the opportunity of counseling couples on coping with the stress of cancer at the University of California Medical Center, San Francisco. In our sessions, I talked with melanoma patients and their spouses about their fears, their beliefs and attitudes, and their plans. I learned that, while fear of death was usually mentioned, concerns about pain, loss of control, and loss of dignity seemed to predominate.

Even in the early stages of cancer, it's important to know that (if it ever becomes necessary) relief from pain is usually possible, that many symptoms can be relieved, and that control and mental clarity can be maintained when medication is skillfully and sensitively administered.

Most patients with cancer will never experience severe pain, but the anticipation of pain causes tension and makes adjusting to the diagnosis even more anxiety provoking. Knowing about the care and effectiveness of hospices and pain clinics has given many patients reassurance that they can be comfortable regardless of the stage of their disease.

If patients mention fear of death, even when the prognosis is favorable, they need to be listened to. Refusal to listen to what may seem like overly negative thinking will only worsen a patient's fears of loss of control and lead him or her to worry in isolation. This unfortunate and all-too-common situation can be avoided by serious talks with the patient of what might be done if the worst happens, and by reassurances from the family and the physician that his or her wishes will be carried out.

Most patients are not afraid of death itself, but fear living their last days in protracted pain with loss of control. Most of those diagnosed with cancer today will never need to look at the last chapter of this book, "Coping with End of Life Issues." Fear of loss of control and a painful death from cancer, however, are so much a part of the fear of the cancer diagnosis that all patients and their loved ones can benefit from learning about what can be done for patients if the disease becomes advanced or terminal.

I know I found it immensely reassuring when, approximately eight years after the diagnosis of my own cancer, I had the opportunity to visit a number of pain clinics and hospices in the United States and England and to see the care that is offered in these centers. The sense of relief and reassurance that I felt made me aware that, even though I have been considered cured of my cancer for several years, I still harbored some dread of dying of cancer in a state of pain, delirium from medication, and loss of control.

Patients and families can reduce their shock from the diagnosis when they realize that not all forms of cancer are terminal. Moreover, in almost every case a clear prognosis cannot be made until tests and treatments show what might work to control, diminish, or completely eradicate the confused cancer cells.

The Stress of the Diagnosis

Patients have reported that the time of the diagnosis was the most stressful part of their cancer experience—more so even than the time of hospitalization and the time before the diagnosis.

The first one hundred days following the diagnosis of cancer have been identified as particularly stressful. During this time, thoughts about life and death predominate, and the patient is more vulnerable to emotional and psychological upset. Those patients who are able to maintain a support network of friends and family, however, are more likely to weather this difficult time without major psychological problems.

When you, the patient, participate in the medical decision-making that will affect your life, some of the stress of the first one hundred days can be alleviated. This spirit of participation is fostered when:

- your feelings, values, and life goals are considered when making medical decisions;

- your opinion and questions are listened to, respected, and answered;

- you are given information about treatment plans and alternatives in a language you can understand;

- both you and the physician are open to negotiating disagreements, rather than maintaining a take-it-or-leave-it attitude.

While the stress, shock, and trauma of the diagnosis and the first months of cancer therapy are intense for most, some comfort can be gathered from knowing that you will most probably find your second hundred days less stressful. This is a time during which you can adjust to your treatment and recovery process. Concerns about life and death issues may continue in your thoughts, but they will give way to the challenges of long-term survival and the small pleasures of living every day more fully.

After coping with the diagnosis and treatment options available to you, you may find that you must adjust your life and career around the scheduling of tests and treatments. The ending of a successful course of treatment and medical appointments leaves some cancer survivors feeling insecure and not quite ready to be on their own again. These feelings can be anticipated and planned for by filling your newly freed-up schedule with more pleasant activities. Follow-up appointments with your doctor should relieve any feelings of abandonment by those who helped you survive a serious threat to your life.

The next stage for most cancer patients involves the challenge of living as a "cancer survivor" and the opportunity to join other survivors on National Cancer Survivors Day (www.ncsdf.org). The National Cancer Institute estimates that in 2003 over 10.5 million Americans had survived cancer. The celebration for cancer survivors and their families takes place on the first Sunday of June in more than 700 locations. To locate the one nearest you, check with the American Cancer Society (www.cancer.org) or contact the National Cancer Survivors Day Foundation at (615) 794-3006 or info@ncsdf.org.

I cannot overestimate the positive impact of seeing hundreds of people who have survived cancer—some who have lived with your type of cancer and your cancer treatments for years and decades. Even if the odds of surviving your type of cancer are not optimistic, you will see, feel, and know the positive, undeniable fact of survival in people like you who overcame those odds and are celebrating their lives.

In 1986, I spoke at a Cancer Survivor Celebration in Walnut Creek, California, and was invited to join a group of twenty-four dedicated people, mostly cancer survivors, to form The National Coalition for Cancer Survivorship (NCCS). NCCS is a wonderful resource for information and support, and serves as an advocate for the employment and insurance rights of cancer survivors. We want to let the world know that there is life after cancer and that cancer survivors have a contribution to make. Information can be found online at www.canceradvocacy.org.

Changes in Self-Perception

If a cancer diagnosis is your first experience of being vulnerable to serious illness, its influence on your self-image can be especially traumatic. You may feel that your body has betrayed you—as if your cells have turned against you. In a very concrete way you realize that you are human and mortal, that life does end, and that your time is limited.

The dramatic change in self-image imposed by cancer is most evident in patients who are teenagers. A cancer diagnosis makes them different from their carefree playmates who seldom believe that the threat of death or even serious illness applies to them. They have not had to face the body's gradual decline that adults begin to experience in their forties or fifties.

Usually they have not seen illness and death strike their peers, so they are unprepared for a life-threatening illness. When it occurs, it shocks them and makes them doubt their underlying assumptions about how the world is supposed to work. But this rapid change in perception can take place in people in their sixties who are accustomed to good health and energy. Some people maintain a teenager's sense of invulnerability and immortality well beyond the age of sixty. For older people whose self-image has remained stable for several decades, a diagnosis of cancer can be dramatically inconsistent with their experience and view of life.

Facing a life-threatening event unites survivors around a new, more realistic view of the world and human courage. It also separates survivors from those who cannot appreciate the cancer experience. Cancer changes not only how you perceive yourself, it changes how others will perceive you and your new attitude toward life and death.

Physicians will treat your physical illness, but you, your family and friends, and your psychosocial counselors will cope with the emotional and psychological changes. You can improve your self-image by accepting mortality and vulnerability to disease as facts for all human beings rather than as signs of personal weakness or failure. A more hardy and realistic self-image will enhance your ability to fight for your life. It will equip you with a better understanding of the social and emotional impact of cancer and will prepare you to cope in ways that contribute to your mental and physical well-being.

Chapter 2

The Power of Your Beliefs

If you had been diagnosed with tuberculosis 150 years ago, the doctors would have told you that you became ill because you are too sensitive and artistic. According to the 1881 edition of *Principles and Practice of Medicine*, the causes of TB were said to be "hereditary disposition, unfavorable climate, sedentary indoor life, defective ventilation, deficiency of light, and depressing emotions." One year later, Robert Koch demonstrated that the primary cause of TB is the tubercle bacillus, for which he won the Nobel Prize in 1905.

The mystery about the causes of cancer leaves us susceptible to a similar tendency to blame the victim and speculating, as people once did with tuberculosis, about a possible defect in personality, thoughts, and attitudes. Today, while medical science continues to make impressive advances into understanding the mechanisms that turn healthy cells into cancerous ones, much remains unknown about what triggers the start of a cancerous growth. Certainly your thoughts and beliefs can affect how you feel, but your conscious mind cannot directly influence the more complex processes such as cell production and removal. Though our knowledge about this relationship remains limited, the press and media continue to speculate about a link between personality type, so-called negative emotions, and disease.

The evidence thus far supports the conclusion that the causes of cancer are primarily biological and not psychological, spiritual, or emotional. However, there are lifestyle changes you can make (see chapter 3) to improve your attitude, the quality of your life, and how well you cope with your illness and medical treatment.

To lower your stress and the tendency to blame yourself for something beyond your control, you might benefit from an examining your beliefs and thoughts about what caused your illness. Do you believe any of the following about your illness? My illness is:

- the result of some sin, bad habit, or a failure to live right

- could have been prevented by doing something different in my life

- is punishment from a vengeful God

- is meant to teach me a lesson

If you hold any of these beliefs or thoughts, how do they affect your ability to cope with medical treatment and possibly help you overcome cancer? This is the real issue, isn't it? You do not need any self-induced stress when you're coping with a serious illness. From a practical standpoint, I recommend that you examine your underlying beliefs and the thoughts that your mind repeats dozens of times a day. Ask yourself these questions:

- What will be the outcome, usefulness, and consequences of continuing to hold the beliefs I learned in the past?

- How do they influence my feelings about myself and my ability to persist in seeking my own survival and happiness?

- Is there one belief that helps lower stress and improve health?

- Can I let go of upsetting beliefs and self-blame in order to accept myself as a human being who has limited control?

- Can will I forgive myself for being human and, therefore, vulnerable to illness, death, and joy?

Why Consider Your Beliefs?

Fighting your own personal battle with cancer is, in many ways, like any other fight for survival—it requires mental toughness, an intense focus on the task, and a refusal to be deterred by the enemy and by your own thoughts. It also requires that you know when to retreat, recover, and recoup your energies for fighting on a better day in another arena. In the course of coping with cancer, you will need to learn how to push away despondency and fears in order to make decisions and take actions that improve your chances of surviving and thriving.

You can benefit from the mental imagery training that peak performing athletes use to prepare themselves for those times when the opponent seems to be winning and when self-doubts abound. Learn to use negative thoughts to remind yourself of the need for a little extra effort, and to turn your focus toward the task, the next step.

You'll want to recognize irrational and unhelpful thoughts and beliefs in order to:

1. Avoid unnecessary feelings of depression and helplessness

2. Formulate positive challenges to negative beliefs

3. Stay committed to coping effectively with cancer and your cancer therapies

4. Maintain a sense of worth and self-respect as a normal human being who is as vulnerable as anyone else to contracting a serious illness

The Meaning of the Word "Cancer"

When the doctor's diagnosis includes the word cancer, the sense of chaos, fear, and loss of control can be so great that you and your family will find it hard to believe what you're hearing. All of a sudden, your trust in an orderly world is shattered and you may be tempted to attribute a special meaning to the disease in order to maintain your expectation of an understandable and controllable world. When horrific events occur, therefore, you may try to explain them in terms of a logical, cause-effect relationship to avoid acknowledging that some things are beyond our human understanding and the control of our medical science.

You may find that you even prefer blame and guilt—with their partially satisfying implication of order and a definite cause—to acceptance of the human condition—with its limited control, unknowable causes, and random victims.

This tendency to deny human vulnerability sometimes leads us to feel anger toward those loved ones who contract a life-threatening disease. They remind us that we too are human, vulnerable, and will die one day. Alice Trillin's article in *The New England Journal of Medicine* poignantly captures a common response to a friend's death:

> I was angry with my friend who died of cancer. I felt that she had let me down, that perhaps she hadn't fought hard enough. It was important for me to find reasons for her death, to find things that she might have done to cause it, as a way of separating myself from her and as a way of thinking that I would somehow have been able to stay alive.

Some part of us wants to believe that if we fight hard enough we should be able to beat cancer. We want to believe that if we had the illness we'd know how to fight and win the battle that our friend has lost. We feel the pull to separate ourselves from loved ones who die and, therefore, from all of humanity in order to hold onto our illusion of invulnerability.

Anger at Yourself for Being Human

When I was a newly diagnosed cancer patient, I did a lot of thinking about my own self-defeating beliefs concerning the causes of cancer and those pressed on me by others. I reminded myself that millions of hypochondriacs, though they believe they have serious illnesses, and constantly are imaging that they are sick, usually live long, healthy lives.

And, of course, even though most of us have felt depressed to the point of thinking about suicide—or at least wanting to put an end to our pain—some life force within us, thankfully, fights to keep us alive in spite of our loss of a will to live. In such moments, we learn that we are not alone. Within us is a force more powerful than our conscious thoughts and feelings of despair and hopelessness. We cannot get through this life struggling alone from the small, fearful parts of ourselves. In the course of a life, we all need to tap into the stronger part of ourselves and seek the support of friends, family, and community to get through many overwhelming challenges.

The Need to Make Sense of Illness and Suffering

Your initial explanation of why you or a loved one contracted a life-threatening illness is an attempt to satisfy your natural need to understand how something so terrible could happen to you and your family.

Holding the popular, but fundamentally flawed belief, that life should always go your way leads to unnecessary pain and anger. If life isn't going the way we think it should be going, we insist that it's going wrong. Someone obviously made a mistake and should be blamed, criticized, and punished.

It is my belief that total, constant health is an ideal, not a constant reality. Though we are capable of robust health most of the time, our bodies coexist on this planet with a multitude of bacteria and viruses; confront numerous stressors, all the while maintaining a delicate internal balance.

Cancer happens. It's not a punishment for wrongdoing or caused by your personality or thoughts. This fact must be borne in mind today, especially when so many movements espouse the doctrine that whatever happens in our lives is under our complete control and chosen by us. Sometimes these beliefs are expressed in a cruel way as when a young man, who was having some difficulty speaking, was introduced to me as, "John, who chose to give himself MS (multiple sclerosis)."

A related school of thought holds that you must admit that you are in part responsible for your disease in order to participate in your healing. Personally, I do not believe that people choose to give themselves MS or cancer, even when they are stressed or depressed. But I do believe that the primary causes of cancer are environmental and biologic, though in some cases—as with tobacco use and a diet high in animal fats—they are linked to our behavior.

Regardless of what started your cancer or caused it to develop at this time, you are still capable of directing your efforts toward recovering from cancer and living a full life, regardless of anyone's theories and beliefs.

Illusion of Control

When we were infants, dependent on our parents for shelter, protection, and food, we couldn't believe that they ever could be imperfect, unstable, or mortal. It was so easy then to make them happy by simply smiling, saying a word or two, or taking our first step. So, of course, we felt powerful and capable of getting what we wanted. It's understandable, therefore, that we cling to what psychologists call "the infant's illusion of omnipotence" and take on inappropriate levels of responsibility for what happens in our families.

A negative side effect of maintaining this illusion is that we hold ourselves responsible for many family problems. From the child's perspective, we'd rather blame ourselves than feel out of control or imagine that our parents might not be powerful enough to keep us from harm.

In times of crisis, we revert to this childlike illusion of control to explain how bad things can happen to good people. It makes us feel more secure to think that we did something wrong rather than accept that we are vulnerable to a world in which cancer and accidents can randomly touch our lives, regardless of how well we live, handle our emotions, or how positive or negative our attitude.

If you deny your human limits, however, you will feel guilty about lacking control over uncontrollable events. Certain phrases in your internal dialogue may reflect a refusal to mourn the loss of the illusion of total control and responsibility. It's not unusual for cancer patients to say to themselves, "You should have known better. If only you had done things differently this wouldn't have happened. It's my fault. How could I sabotage myself this way?" Statements such as these are symptoms of being stuck in a fantasy about how life should be and of not knowing how to let go of the illusion of unlimited power.

As an attempt to explain uncontrollable events, blame and self-criticism are particularly damaging to your ability to cope with cancer. Self-blame for having cancer can result in feelings of depression that contribute to delays in seeking medical treatment, inhibitions about discussing feelings and concerns, and a diminished ability to form helpful relationships with doctors, social workers, and family members. Realistically accepting your human vulnerability to illness, however, can help you alleviate unnecessary guilt and self-blame and turn your energies toward coping more effectively in those areas where you do have some control over how you cope.

How You Try to Explain Suffering

The strength and compassion of religious and spiritual beliefs are tested by the physical, psychological, and emotional stress of cancer. You may want to re-examine your beliefs if they contribute to feelings of guilt rather than serve to comfort you. In *When Bad Things Happen to Good People*, Rabbi Harold Kushner writes of his message to a young man in his community who was dying of a degenerative disease:

I don't know why my friend and neighbor is sick and dying and in constant pain. From my religious perspective, I cannot tell him that God has His reasons for sending him this terrible fate, or that God must specially love him or admire his bravery to test him in this way. I can only tell him that the God I believe in did not send the disease and does not have a miraculous cure that He is withholding.

In his attempt to understand how bad things can happen to good people, Rabbi Kushner concludes that the laws of nature impact all alike and that not even God interferes with these laws.

Any beliefs that lead you to think of cancer as punishment from God should be examined carefully with the help of clergy or counselors. Personal and spiritual beliefs that accept human suffering as a natural part of life and facilitate forgiveness for being vulnerable human beings are more likely to assist rapid adaptation to illness and even lead to spiritual transformation.

Review Your Reactions to the Diagnosis

Initially, it may be hard to remember how you reacted and what beliefs you clung to when you first heard the diagnosis of cancer. The shock and numbing effect upon hearing any bad news has its purposes. It allows us to carry on while our brain begins to make sense of the implications of what we've been through. In the long run, however, it usually makes sense to be consciously aware of what you have to deal with and examine your initial reactions in order to:

1. Correct those initial reactions and misinterpretations which may be keeping you stuck in persistent worries and upsetting emotions

2. Identify those areas for which you need more information or clearer communication

3. Have a common starting point from which you can share

your reactions, observations, and feelings with your family and friends

4. Learn that others are more perceptive than you imagined—for instance, they saw through your brave facade

5. Alleviate the trauma of those initial stresses by seeing them from a new perspective

If your memory of your initial reactions needs jogging, you may want to go through the "Exercise for Recall of the Diagnosis" in appendix A and then complete reading the rest of this section.

As you think of the time of the diagnosis, what thoughts, feelings, attitudes, and beliefs do you become aware of?

- Are you surprised to learn of reactions and ideas or events that you didn't remember? Shock and numbness can cause you to miss what's being said.

- How does your memory of the diagnosis match that of your family or your doctor?

- What did they think of how you were feeling and coping?

- What were your thoughts about them and their concerns?

You'll find that if you simply observe what happened, rather than judge it, you will become aware of more and more. When reexamining their feelings at that time, many people find that one of their first reactions upon hearing the diagnosis was to assume that they will soon die; this reaction reveals to them their underlying belief that having cancer must automatically mean death. Many find themselves thinking:

- I have cancer. I'm going to die.

- Why me? Why now?

- This shouldn't be happening. I can't believe it.

- What did I do to deserve this?

- Why would God want to give me cancer?

- What am I supposed to learn?

Others become aware of their anger at their doctor for the way in which the news was presented, or simply for bringing them bad news. Others learn that they blotted out any emotional reactions for a time and quickly occupied themselves with gathering data. It's not unusual for people to feel a sense of relief on hearing the diagnosis—relief at finally knowing what is wrong.

All of these reactions are legitimate and, regardless of which reactions you had, don't judge them. Given the information you had and your needs at the time, you coped as best you could. Now the job is to examine those attitudes and beliefs that persist to determine whether they continue to serve you. If they do not, update them with new styles of coping that fit your current situation and give you energy to maximize your joy and minimize your sadness.

New Ways of Thinking about Cancer

Dealing with cancer is going to tax your resources to the limit, and you will find it beneficial to learn new ways of looking at your experience and at life in general.

Start by examining your reactions to your diagnosis and share this experience with those close to you. As you think about your experience, you will notice, certain statements or feelings appear repeatedly. These statements reveal the underlying beliefs and concepts that influence your current actions. Many of them may be erroneous; some are simply outdated; others are partially true, and some may be very accurate. Before you get overcommitted to any of these beliefs, you may want to examine how your beliefs, and their underlying meaning, affect you emotionally and behaviorally.

Let's look at ways to challenge or replace some of the common stressful reactions to hearing a diagnosis of cancer.

Five Stressful Reactions

Stressful Reaction 1—Why me?

"Why me?" or its variant, "Why now?" imply that what happened shouldn't have happened, is unfair, or that something or somebody is to blame.

While many think this is the usual reaction to a cancer diagnosis, I have worked with several patients for whom "Why not me?" was more natural. Betty Rollins was a cancer patient who, when she saw others suffer, would ask herself, "Why should they suffer? Why them? Why not me?" In writing about her experience with breast cancer, she states, "I felt that losing a breast was lousy, but I never felt that losing a breast was unfair." Rollins' question is the more compassionate one that asks, "Why should anyone suffer pain, illness, or death?"

The question "Why?" often implies guilt and blame, as when we ask a child, "Why did you spill the milk?" Such a question accuses the child of consciously plotting to spill the milk and of being aware of his or her motives. Some would go so far as to suggest that the child has an unconscious motive such as hostility or vengeance.

Blaming and analyzing leads to faulty theorizing, a failure to offer directions on how to clean up the mess, and little room for the necessary trial-and-error learning on the part of a child whose muscles and body are growing and changing every week. In fact, the emotional upset and mental confusion caused by trying to answer the irrelevant question "Why" only adds to a sense of failure and self-blame and lessens the child's ability to learn new behavior and take corrective action.

Having cancer is difficult enough without adding to it guilt and concern that something may be wrong with you as a person. "Why me?" or "Why did this have to happen now?" are not very useful questions, unless you want to feel guilty and confused. You will find it much more effective to rapidly replace such thoughts with responses such as: "What can I do about it now?" "This time, it is me that it happened to." "Yes, it's difficult, lousy, bad timing, and unfair, but now that it has happened, what can I do to adjust and to improve my chances of survival?"

These last statements quickly get you beyond the frustrating and ineffectual thoughts like, "What did I do to deserve this?" and "This shouldn't have happened," to acknowledging that it did happen. Now is the time for action and for focusing your brain on taking major steps toward solving problems and less stressful ways of coping.

Stressful Reaction 2—It's God's will that I have cancer.

This statement may be comforting to those who believe that God has chosen them to carry out a difficult assignment for some unexplained reason. From this point of view, cancer can be seen as an opportunity to learn something important from the experience.

Some, however, may interpret this statement to mean that God is punishing them for something that they did or failed to do. This interpretation is most regrettable and can cause unnecessary grief and despair.

Others, like my uncle Pat, choose to see cancer, suffering, pain, and death as natural parts of life. When Uncle Pat had painful cancer of the intestine, I asked this wonderfully accepting and religious man about how he made sense of how God worked. He answered:

> Let me tell you a story. One day God sent St. Peter down to Earth to see how things were going. St. Peter returned to Heaven very upset, and in a complaining tone he told God, "Nothing is fair down there. There is suffering and pain; some are healthy and others are ill. It's so unfair! Nothing is the way it should be." God looked at St. Peter with patience and understanding and said, "No Peter, everything is just as it should be. Everything is fine."

If you find yourself committed to the belief that cancer is God's will, you might try going beyond the usual interpretation of painful events as punishment and consider illness, pain, and death as natural to this world—neither good or bad. You might wonder, with a great sense of curiosity, how the support of resources—deep within you—will help you to make something of this experience.

Stressful Reaction 3—I made a mistake. If I lived differently, I wouldn't have cancer.

As with the statement, "Why me?" these phrases imply that things should or could be different. But they also may have a specific behavior to point to, such as smoking, drinking, or working in an asbestos plant. The problem with such thoughts is that they can keep you endlessly brooding over the past without taking any corrective action.

You now have knowledge that you didn't have back then. You're smarter and will continue to get smarter as you go through life. It's like the process of climbing a mountain—as you climb, you gain a clearer view of where you're going and which path will get you there. You would be foolish to plan the entire ascent from the base of the mountain. You can plan the basic approach to your climb, but the specific steps can only be chosen alone the way, requiring revisions at each plateau, as you gain more knowledge.

If you confront a crevasse that was not visible from the base of the mountain, did you make a mistake? Should you chastise yourself for being foolish or ill-informed? Or can you include this new information in your plans and proceed on your journey, even if you must backtrack a bit? We certainly don't consider amendments to the Constitution of the United States as mistakes made by the Founding Fathers. In fact, the strength of the Constitution comes from its ability to allow for changes that require the continual inclusion of new information and the agonizing processes of adjustment. These changes and adjustments are not mistakes. They are realistic confrontations with the facts of life as they are today. The more rapidly you acknowledge and accept today's facts, the more rapidly you can make the necessary changes and maximize your experience.

As you focus on what you can do now, your mind will shift from past events—which you are helpless to change—to problem solving in the present, the only time in which you can be effective.

Stressful Reaction 4—Cancer is terminal. I'm going to die.

This belief has frightened patients away from seeking a diagnosis and from following through on medical treatments that could save their lives. Without knowing your unique circumstances, it is difficult to challenge this belief without sounding trite and overly optimistic. But I will take that risk because I know that you can learn to constructively challenge and replace your initial, distressing thoughts with direct statements of today's facts.

First, more than sixty-five percent of all cancers today are curable, and ninety percent of many forms of cancer are curable or can be held in remission. Second, many people can live with cancer for many productive and enjoyable years. Third, the diagnosis of cancer does not mean that you will die immediately, nor does it mean that you will ever die of cancer.

If you are like most of us who have been diagnosed with a life-threatening illness, you may have never thought about the possibility of dying. But now you may be dealing with the unwelcome prospect of dying earlier than you anticipated. The simple fact is that all of us will die someday, but most of us never use that fact to enrich our lives.

At one of the yearly Cancer Survivor Celebrations—held on the first Sunday in June—a cancer survivor said, "We are among those initiated to the facts of life. We say *when* I die as opposed to the uninitiated who say *if* I die." As one of those initiated to the realities of human life, you have an opportunity to make your life richer and of higher quality than before, because you now know that life is a precious, limited resource to be experienced fully each moment with a clear and honest expression of your feelings.

I met a seventy-two year-old woman who told me that in her

youth, she was very careful with her money because she was frightened of being homeless when she reached old age. She worried about the future and never spent a cent on pleasurable activities. Early in her forties—at a time when treatments options were limited—she contracted breast cancer and realized that she might never have a chance to get old. She told herself, "This is *my* old age."

With the very real probability of death before her, she decided that she could now spend the money that she was saving for her old age. After her surgery she planned and took her first trip around the world. Faced with what she believed to be a much shorter lifespan, she started enjoying life rather than trying to protect it for some imagined future that might never happen. Her cancer diagnosis completely changed her outlook on life.

To her amazement, she lived a long, adventurous, and productive life into her nineties and took more than nineteen trips around the world.

Stressful Reaction 5—Cancer is powerful, and my body is weak and defenseless.

When I first got cancer I wanted to literally fight it. I wanted to smash it as if it were an insect. And later, when friends and family members contracted cancer, I felt the same way, frustrated that cancer seemed too intangible to fight. It was part of the very cells of our bodies and could not be grappled with as an enemy separate from the person.

And, the commonly accepted notion that "cancer spreads to your lungs and lymph nodes" only adds to feeling too helpless to do anything. It gives you the false image that your body is passive and cancer is powerful. In fact, your lungs filter the blood of debris, and your lymph nodes hold bacteria and cancer cells. Your body is active in the fight against cancer.

You may find it more helpful, and more accurate, to think of cancer cells as having a confused nucleus and to imagine how cancer therapy destroys these confused cells by taking advantage of their inability to reproduce when exposed to certain chemical agents and radiation. Your healthy hair and mucous membrane cells, however, will recover.

The body routinely develops precancerous cells, identifies them, and destroys them. The body is quite powerful in the face of cancer. Every day we are learning more about the ability of the immune system to identify, destroy, and remove dying cells, foreign matter, and debris. We are just learning from discoveries about the ability of scavenger cells called macrophages to selectively identify tumor cells, ingest them, and release an enzyme that attacks them.

Begin thinking, "My body is strong and capable of cooperating with medical treatment to eliminate cancer cells." Yes, cancer needs to be taken seriously and to be treated with strong medical procedures. But remember to acknowledge that most of your body has strong, healthy cells that will recover from these powerful medicines, and can use its many defenses to help in the fight against cancer.

Where Do I Go From Here?

You'll find it helpful to continually challenge any negative thoughts and beliefs with realistic and positive thoughts that give you hope and optimize your chances of survival. Replace theorizing about the causes of cancer with thoughts that give you a positive focus such as, "Where do I go from here?" and "What can I do now?"

Notice which beliefs prepare you to actively participate in your cancer therapy and help you improve your relationships with your doctors, nurses, family, and friends. Identify those beliefs that mobilize your physical and mental energies to optimize your chances to overcome cancer.

While the tendency to have thoughts of self-blame—even for events out of your control—is a typical initial reaction, it can waste your valuable time and energy. You can't change the past or control the future. The fact is that you can work only in the present, from where you are now, with what you know now, and with the resources you have now. A more effective statement, therefore, is, "How do I deal with my current situation? I'm committed to taking whatever small steps I can to improve my life and my ability to cope with this illness."

It is my belief that most cancers can be beaten while many more can be lived with for years. With the help of medical treatments to lessen the tumor load, your body has the ability to identify and remove the remaining microscopic cancer cells that are less than one percent of your entire body.

As you challenge your initial reactions and former beliefs they will give way to a more thoughtful consideration of what you can do now to cope most effectively with the journey ahead of you.

Chapter 3

Maintaining a Fighting Spirit: What You Can Do

When you've been diagnosed with cancer, the doctor's job of removing the malignant cells from your body is the top priority. This part of the mission to save your life usually involves surgery and chemotherapy or radiation. But you, as a member of the healthcare team, have an essential part to play in carrying out this mission. With the support of your doctor and nutritionist, you can make changes in diet, exercise, and health habits that could improve your body's ability to adapt to your medical treatments and increase your chances of returning to full health.

It may seem too late to make lifestyle changes after you've been diagnosed with cancer, but there are things you can do to optimize your body's ability to cooperate with cancer-fighting medicines and to contain and remove cancerous cells.

How to Reduce Stress During a Stressful Time

In my thirty years of preparing patients for surgery, chemotherapy, and radiation, I have observed that reducing stress enables patients to recover more rapidly, and with less pain, than the doctors predict. Keep in mind that my conclusions are based not on stringent research—which would include control groups—but on the self-reports of my clients recovering from major cancer surgeries—as well hip, knee, and shoulder surgeries—and chemotherapy and radiation treatment.

As part of their preparation, I give my clients the positive suggestion that the body knows how to recover from surgery and wounds and can cooperate with chemo- and radiation therapies to remove the confused cancer cells. I also recommend the methods listed below.

Five Actions to Make More Energy Available for Healing

> *Important Note: The suggestions made here and elsewhere in this book are not meant to replace the recommendations of your doctors or other healthcare professionals.*

Since receiving a "terminal" cancer diagnosis in 1974—and pronounced cured after surgery and extensive chemotherapy—I've worked with cancer patients, their families, and with oncology departments across the country. From my clinical work with hundreds of patients with serious illnesses, and what I've learned from the research literature, I've concluded that five activities seem to help many reduce stress, improve attitude, and possibly strengthen immune system response. You might try one or more that suit your style and your needs.

1. Express Honest Emotions

Express your emotions honestly, especially the more difficult emotions of anger and sadness, rather than trying to be stoic or falsely cheerful.

Write or record your feelings and thoughts every day for at least fifteen minutes, or speak to a therapist or member of the clergy once a week. Don't ruminate about difficulties for more than a few hours before expressing them to someone or writing them out. Shout them in your car. Sing the blues. Dance or walk with a vengeance. Get those feelings out of your gut-level response and put them into words and movement.

For more regarding the impressive research on how writing about your feelings can improve the strength of your immune system, see Dr. James W. Pennebaker's *Opening Up: The Healing Power of Expressing Emotions.*

Tell yourself, "I can accept your emotions. They don't scare me. I accept you even though you feel angry or depressed."

Use a form of "self-talk" in which you, from your highest self and values, conduct a dialogue with the overwhelmed, frightened parts of yourself. You then take on the leadership and protective roles that empower you to speak up and stand up for your body and life.

2. Create Safety to Lower Stress

Practice meditative or relaxation exercises for stress and pain reduction. These can help soften the impact of negative messages and challenging events.

Take three slow, deep breaths—inhale, hold, exhale slowly and float down into the support of chair and floor. Close your eyes and let go of muscle tension as your body and mind connect with a larger support system in my brain and body. Remind yourself that all around you is a protective atmosphere weighing at least fourteen pounds per square inch—thick enough to burn up most meteorites before they reach you. You might imagine this atmosphere as a white or golden bubble of light three to four feet all around you, protecting you from the noises outside and giving you all the time in the world to push aside any concerns or unwanted thoughts; all the time in the world to keep yourself safe and calm.

Tell yourself, "This event is not the end of the world. This is only a 3.0, not a 10.0-level earthquake or tornado. Regardless of what happens, your worth as a person is safe with me. I won't let this ruin my evening. I won't make you feel bad."

3. Shift from Worry to Wonder

Maintain a sense of wonder about how your body will work with medical treatment and will use its own wisdom to heal and create greater comfort.

Practice shifting from worry to wonder. Use any sign of worry—holding your breath, muscle tension, tightening your jaw, fist, or forehead—to remind you to let go of holding on and to delegate that energy to the superior wisdom of your body, your Inner Healer, and your Inner Physician. Be honest about your fears and worries but do not assume that your conscious mind's worries are the whole picture. Regardless of the statistics you were told, remember that no one can predict your odds of survival. You are a unique individual, not a statistic. Maintain a sense of wonder. Expect a positive surprise.

Tell yourself, "This is going to be interesting. I wonder how the wisdom in my body and brain will help me get through this. I wonder what resources my body and mind will access."

4. Choose Your Treatment

Maintain some control over medical decisions, seek second and third opinions, ask questions of your doctor, and decide what you will do—for example, exercise and diet and meditation or prayer—that could enhance the effects of medical treatment and strengthen your body.

Refuse to make yourself feel like a victim by repeating "I have to take chemotherapy" or, "I have to go into surgery." Choosing to do what makes sense will help you break through ambivalence and inner conflict and will calm your mind and soothe your body. Remember, your ability to choose is what makes you human. It is a third place beyond the inner conflict and ambivalence of "You have to" versus "I don't want to."

Tell yourself, "I can choose to do what increases my chances of survival. You do not *have to* get surgery, chemotherapy, or radiation. And, you don't have to want to take these treatments. I, your higher brain and higher Self, can *choose* to do what is difficult but essential for survival."

5. Let Go of the Past

Mourn your losses and adapt to the present condition, rather than struggling to change the past.

Replace all "should've" and "could've" thoughts about the past with what you can do now. Catch your mind drifting into the past and bring it back to maximize the pleasure of the present moment and what you can do now that is consistent with your current goals.

Tell yourself: "That was awful. It really hurt. It's over. And I can choose what to do now to minimize my pain and maximize my joy."

Practice these five activities and adapt them to your style and beliefs and you will most likely find that you feel less stressed, more in control, and grateful to gain the cooperation of your mind and body in this battle to beat cancer.

Expect a Surprise

When doctors observe how patients using these methods recover from surgery so quickly, with minimal discomfort, they often use words such as "amazed," "astonished," and "surprised." As a result, I now ask my clients—as part of their positive suggestions—to bring back to me the doctor's message of surprise at how easily they underwent surgery and how rapidly they recovered. And most are successful at amazing their doctors with their rapid recovery.

Of course, I cannot guarantee that these methods will work as well for everyone, but they are worth considering as ways of lowering stress and making your unique contribution to coping with this serious illness.

(See chapter 4 to learn in greater detail how to manage your stress during this most stressful of times.)

Replace Negative Reactions

You can develop a more helpful attitude for coping with cancer by examining your initial reactions to your diagnosis and the beliefs that underlie them. Here are some common negative reactions to cancer and some suggestions for useful responses to replace them.

Negative Reaction: Why me? Why now? Life is unfair.

Healthy Response: Now that it has happened and it is me, what can I do about it? As awful as this situation is, what can I do to improve my chances of beating cancer?

Negative Reaction: Cancer is powerful, and my body is weak. Cancer means death.

Healthy Response: Cancer cells are, in fact, abnormal cells that are weak. These confused cells cannot reproduce when exposed to chemotherapy or radiation. My immune system routinely identifies and destroys malformed cells and removes them from my body. My body can cooperate with medical treatment in destroying and removing cancer cells.

Negative Reaction: If I had lived life differently, I wouldn't have cancer. I wish I could do it over again.

Healthy Response: The past is over, and I cannot control it or change it. It did happen. It does hurt. But I do have control over how I make myself feel in the present. I am focusing on what I can do now.

Make note of any repeated thoughts that leave you feeling down and self-critical. Develop challenges to these thoughts that focus your mind on what you can do now and on helpful images of coping in the future.

Nutrition: Feeding the Healthy Part of You

Much of the information listed here was gathered from the National Cancer Institute (NCI) website, http:// cancer.gov, and the American Cancer Society's site,

> *www.cancer.org. For the most current information,*
> *visit these sites or call NCI at 1-800-4-CANCER or the*
> *American Cancer Society at 1-800-ACS-2345.*

I'm not expert in nutrition or the correlation between diet and cancer, so I can't give you advice about what you should or shouldn't eat. I've learned that supplements, foods, and activities that a majority of people find helpful can still be detrimental to certain individuals and conditions. So, check with your doctor before making any dietary changes and always honor your own body's reactions.

That said, I can tell you what dietary changes I made to facilitate my body's adjustment to chemotherapy. When I started chemo, I knew that I was asking my body to tolerate strong chemicals that could kill and remove cancer cells and that also could do some temporary harm to my liver, hair, and mucous membranes. To assist my body in rapidly digesting and eliminating possible toxins, therefore, I tripled my daily intake of vegetables and fruits, ate fresh fish at least once a week, and stopped eating red and processed meats for nine months

I made sure that cruciferous vegetables such as broccoli and cauliflower were included in my meals because their high levels of antioxidants have been found to inhibit the growth of cancer cells, and they are linked to a lower risk of cancer. (For more information about the benefits of diet and physical activity see the American Cancer Society's contact information above.)

Later, I learned that the apples, onions, garlic, tea, red grapes, berries, broccoli, and leafy greens I added to my diet contain the helpful antioxidants called bioflavonoid, which are one of the body's mechanisms for inhibiting tumor growth. Today, I continue to maintain a healthy diet and exercise program but will have a few meals each year that contain red or processed meats. I've learned to enjoy finding creative ways of preparing vegetables, salads, and whole grains, and I keep a bowl of apples, oranges, bananas, jicama, or berries available in my kitchen for snacks and dessert.

In addition to these dietary and lifestyle changes, I practiced the five activities mentioned above to make more energy available for healing. I expressed, verbally and in writing, my honest emotions and was fortunate enough to have the opportunity to use my experience to help others. I highly recommend that you write out your feelings and, if it feels comfortable for you, join a support group for patients and survivors such as those offered by I Can Cope, the Wellness Community, and the National Coalition for Cancer Survivorship. These groups will offer you the opportunity to express your feelings and to share your experiences with other patients and survivors.

One doctor told me that because cancer motivated me to improve my diet and change my former "Type A" behavior, I probably avoided having a heart attack by age fifty.

Nutrition Research

The jury is still out on what changes in diet will increase your chances of survival once you've been diagnosed with cancer, but recent studies point toward several things you can do to lower the risk of life-threatening illnesses such as cancer and heart disease.

The following have been found to be associated with living a longer, healthier, and more robust life:

- stop smoking

- lose weight if you are overweight

- exercise—10 to 30 minutes of walking a day is adequate

- decrease the amount of red and processed meats—limit to once or twice a week

- eat more vegetables and fruit—five portions a day—especially the cruciferous vegetables like broccoli, cauliflower, Brussel sprouts, and cabbage. They are high in fiber and help you excrete excess estrogen.

- eat more whole grains and dietary fibers

"The basics of good nutrition have not changed." wrote Jane

Brody, in her January 1, 2008 *New York Times* column. "Meals replete with vegetables, fruits and whole grains and a small serving of a protein-rich food remain the gold standard of a wholesome diet." Brody further states that in 2007 the American Institute for Cancer Research in conjunction with the World Cancer Research Fund published a report based on 7,000 studies of seventeen kinds of cancer. It concluded that:

- smoking and being overweight are the top two preventable causes of cancer;

- frequent consumption of red and processed meats is associated with an increased risk for colon and rectal cancer;

- there's "convincing evidence" for physical activity offering some protection against colon and rectal cancers; and,

- consumption of dietary fibers, nonstarchy vegetables, fruits, folates, beta-carotene, vitamin C, selenium, milk, and calcium supplements (limiting to 1000 milligrams) offers "probable" protection against a variety of cancers.

Race and Cancer

Early detection and early treatment is essential in reducing the risk of fatal cancers regardless of your racial or ethnic background. African-American women, however, have a 10 percent lower rate of breast cancer than white women, yet they die of this cancer at a higher rate. Young black women are especially vulnerable to the most aggressive forms of cancer. The higher rate of cancer mortality among black women is due in part to less medical insurance, fewer routine mammograms, and reduced access to the latest cancer treatments.

For information on support for black women with cancer, see www.sistersnetworkinc.org or call 866/781-1808. You can email them at infonet@sistersnetworkinc.org.

Too Much of a Good Thing

One of the lessons we've learned from reading about fad diets and so-called "miracle supplements" is that we need to see the results of long-term studies before we go overboard. Be careful about taking massive doses of any supplement. Inform your doctor of all over-the-counter supplements or medications. Some of these may, for example, thin your blood or interact with prescribed medications. Keep within the recommended doses of any multivitamin-mineral supplement, and stay on a diet high in vegetables and fruits.

Not everything is good for everybody. While many foods are not hazardous when consumed in moderation, breast cancer patients, for example, may need to avoid soy supplements. Excessive amounts of vitamins A, B6, B12, C, E, and K, or niacin, folic acid, calcium, magnesium, iron, and zinc can lead to complications when combined with prescription medicines, homeopathic remedies, and over-the-counter medications.

Expect a Positive Transformation

Any crisis offers an opportunity for positive change, and for many cancer patients coping with the diagnosis and treatment of cancer calls forth a transformation in attitude, health habits, and self-image. Facing a life-threatening experience stretches your abilities beyond previously accepted limits and gives you a chance to achieve your greatest potential. In a crisis, you must replace ineffective and limited ways of coping and replace them with healthier methods of working and relating.

In short, the cancer experience holds the possibility of making your life more focused, mindful, and meaningful. Learning to make lifestyle changes in attitude, health habits, and in managing stress and social pressures can prepare you to cope more effectively with cancer and lead to a fuller life after cancer.

Chapter 4

Managing the Stress of Serious Illness

The stress of cancer and cancer treatment can be physical, emotional, and social. Your strategies for coping with cancer, therefore, can include ways to calm your physical stress response, restore a sense of emotional control, and help you maintain strength in your relationships. With practice almost everyone—regardless of age, education, or personality—can learn to lower his or her stress hormones within thirty seconds.

All the patients who used the methods you'll be learning in this chapter have achieved some measure of relaxation and calm. Many, but not all, achieve dramatic results such as maintaining a calm state of mind, recovering rapidly from treatments, and managing pain, nausea, and insomnia. At the very least, you can expect to learn how to calm your heart rate, release muscle tension, and feel a sense of relief within minutes. That alone is quite an achievement and of much benefit, physically and psychologically. When you learn to shut off your stress response, you'll be exercising skills at communicating with, and gaining the cooperation of, your mind and body.

These tools will put you in charge of your stress response and will, therefore, facilitate your recuperation, healing, and peace of mind.

Understanding Your Healthy Stress Response

The following five major concepts about stress, distress, and stress management will give you a new perspective on your body's healthy survival response and help you manage the emotional and physical impact of cancer.

1. Your Survival Response

What people are usually referring to when they speak of feeling *stress* is actually a natural survival *response*. This *stress response* takes place when the body reacts to signs of danger—whether from external threats or self-threats of anger and pressure. This natural survival response includes activating the adrenal glands, constricting blood vessels, and raising blood pressure to rush blood to the heart, brain, and large muscles. The heart rate is increased, the clotting response is accelerated, the immune response is put on alert, and, in extreme cases, the stomach and bowels will be cleared.

The stress response rushes blood away from the extremities toward the more essential organs, leaving the palms cool and then damp. Adrenaline makes the heart beat faster, and you may experience butterflies in the stomach because the processes of digestion and elimination are halted to conserve energy for survival. All of this takes place when your brain receives a message of danger and prepares your body for the fight-or-flight survival response.

2. Distress

Distress occurs when you use this survival response repeatedly with no chance to direct the tremendous burst of energy that has been called forth, and with no time to recuperate. During a stress response, the body produces a multitude of hormones to prepare your muscles for battle or escape. These preparations would be extremely useful if you were confronting a tangible, physical threat you could fight or run away from.

In a physical fight for survival, you use these hormones as they were intended, working your muscles, releasing muscle tension, and leaving you exhausted and ready for deep sleep and recovery. But when the struggle is mental, or involves images of future battles, your body builds up energy that cannot be directed toward any target. This disrupts the normal cycle of hormone release, use, and then rest, causing adrenal fatigue and distress.

The results of distress can be seen in "battle fatigue" in which soldiers are continually stressed with little opportunity to experience periods of safety, rest, and recuperation. But the more common forms of distress come from threats to our self-worth, threats from imagined catastrophes, or from our own conflicting messages.

3. Stressful Beliefs

The belief that you must feel upset if something unpleasant happens to you, or if you fail to achieve what you want, will make you more vulnerable to distress. Such beliefs insinuate that negative events must lead you to feel undeserving of happiness, to lose self-esteem, and may cause you to threaten yourself with self-hatred—the ultimate source of self-induced stress.

Conversely, if you believe in your innate worth and that life usually includes painful events that have nothing to do with your worth or goodness, you can manage these events with minimal stress. Your coping will actually be more effective because you focus on problem solving rather than the self-criticism and self-hatred that triggers a stress response. Maintaining self-worth, regardless of what happens means that you will call forth the appropriate levels of energy to take action rather than the high levels of stress hormones needed to defend yourself.

4. Stuck Energy

Your nervous system responds to your thoughts and images as if they are real and happening now. There is no past or future for the nervous system. There is only now. Distress and anxiety occur when you create images of past events or worry about potential problems you anticipate in an imagined future time.

These images provoke energy that can't be used now, leaving you feeling stuck with anxiety. Once you focus your attention on what you can do now, your body releases this stuck energy and you experience excitement, productivity, and effectiveness.

When you give your body a clear message about what to do now in the real time of this moment, you'll eliminate anxiety, lower stress, and become infinitely more productive.

If it could speak, your distressed, overwhelmed body might ask:

- What level of stress and energy do you need for this task?

- Are we fighting a tiger or sitting still for an injection?

- Are you just worrying about potential problems in the future, feeling guilty about past behavior, or is there something I can work on now?

To treat this faithful servant with respect you must repeatedly

The Power of Imagery

Though your body and brain have vast subconscious resources—and a wisdom that includes knowledge for your survival and joyful living—you probably limit your identity to just the conscious part of you. But you can learn to expand your identity to access these resources and communicate with your body and brain in clear images that elicit the levels of energy that are consistent with your health and goals.

Your body is a faithful servant that responds to the images you and your environment present to it. As you read the following passage, notice how your body responds to the images.

Imagine that you are in a garden. The green grass, trees, and flowers present you with a quiet, peaceful feeling. Not far away is a lush lemon tree, heavy with bright, yellow lemons that contrast with its deep green leaves. As you approach this tree, your attention is drawn to a particularly large, ripe lemon. You reach for it, pluck it, bring your time-traveling mind into the present so your body can release the energy you called for.

As you practice living in the present moment, you will lower both anxiety and stress and, therefore, improve your body's ability to work with medical treatments.

5. *You Don't Have to Struggle Alone*

Though the body has its limits, it possesses wisdom that is far beyond the abilities of your conscious mind. Your autonomic nervous system, cells, molecules, atoms, and subatomic photons and protons contain a wisdom that far surpasses that of your central nervous system and consciously controlled muscles.

---

and take a closer look. You can see and feel the pitted texture of its skin. You now grasp it firmly and cut it open, watching as the juice begins to flow. The fragrance of fresh lemon is in the air. As you bring the freshly cut lemon closer, and prepare to bite into it, you become aware that your body has already prepared you for the tartness of the lemon's juice.

Observe how your body prepares to respond to the images you have given it. You might prefer to think about your favorite holiday meal or vacation spot, and find that this image produces an even more powerful and more pleasurable effect. But your body will also respond to images of worry, guilt, or messages of threat or self-hatred with a stress response that prepares you for a catastrophe and danger.

It makes sense, therefore, to appreciate your body's protective survival response and to be careful of the images and messages you give yourself. Your brain and body will also respond to messages of safety by shutting off the stress response and the stress hormones, allowing you to heal more quickly.

You and your conscious mind don't have to struggle alone when you can learn to access your right brain, subconscious, autonomic genius that resides deep within you. While you are sitting there, reading this book, and continuing to breathe normally and regularly, without thinking about it, you are making millions of healthy new cells every minute. Each week you make new hair, nails, skin cells, and a new lining to your esophagus.

And you don't have to know how to make even one cell. Yet the wiser part of you knows more than modern science about making cells, removing malformed cells, and fighting viruses and bacteria. Your subconscious mind knows a lot more than your conscious mind will ever know. The physical part of you performs countless miracles for your survival every second. You never have to stress yourself about this. The conscious part of you can let go of struggling alone and can exhale to discover that you have a larger, wiser support system within.

Regaining Physical Control

You can use stress management techniques to gain physical control over a body whose very cells seem to have gone awry, to gain mental control over the flood of distressing and counterproductive thoughts and images, and to assert your worth in an environment of strong social pressures.

Serious illness is often experienced as a loss of control over your body and life—loss to both the illness and its medical treatment. The ability to relax deeply, to experience a washing away of tension, and to feel that your own body can still provide pleasure and rest, is a powerful sign of hope for any patient facing a life-threatening illness. Gaining even minimal control of your body's reactions will restore a sense of harmonious functioning that can revitalize your connection with your body.

A number of methods are available for relaxing the body and providing some comfort for most patients: listening to music, warm baths, massage, exercise, meditation, autogenic training, self-hypnosis, biofeedback, and yoga. I have found the following exercise, adapted from the Menninger Clinic's Autogenic Exercise, effective with many patients and their family members.

Talking to Your Body

This is an exercise for taking charge of or influencing body functions, such as blood flow to warm your hands, by using a language that your body can cooperate with.

Through this exercise, you learn to use *passive volition* to communicate in words and images that produce relaxation, recovery from fatigue, and improved circulation.

In this first stage of gaining physical control through relaxation, you can achieve adequate levels of relaxation with increasingly beneficial results within a week or two of daily practice sessions of ten to fifteen minutes. It's important that you resist the urge to test out your new skills during the most stressful events in your life until you experience effective self-soothing and relaxation in normal settings.

You may want to make an audio recording of this exercise starting here. Listening to this exercise in your own voice can bring about profound relaxation.

This self-control exercise is directed toward warming your hands and relaxing your entire body. You can only achieve this by letting go of conscious attempts at control and by allowing the automatic part of your nervous system do its job.

In doing this exercise, you will be accomplishing the amazing feat of dilating the blood vessels and capillaries in your hands and fingers. You cannot accomplish this by commanding it to happen, the way you might if you wanted to open your hand. You can only accomplish this by learning to speak in a language that your subconscious mind understands, and by trusting in your inner wisdom to bring you deep relaxation and rapid recuperation for your own health and benefit.

Start by sitting upright in a chair with your feet flat on the floor and your hands on your thighs. Inhale deeply, hold your breath for a moment, and then exhale slowly and completely. Do this three times, counting each time you exhale. Let each exhalation be a signal that you are letting go of any remaining tension.

Now allow your eyelids to close softly. You may try to keep them open and find that it's much more comfortable to allow them to float softly down over your eyes.

Allow the relaxation to flow down over your entire body. Now shift your attention to the chair. Let yourself float down into the chair. Let the chair, the floor, or the bed support you. Let go of any unnecessary tension in your muscles. Shift your attention to the floor, and let it support your feet. Now you can let go of those muscles. As you let go, continue to exhale away any remaining tension.

During these next few minutes, there's nothing much for you to do except to allow your conscious mind to be curious as your body and subconscious mind cooperate with the process of providing you deeper and deeper relaxation with each phrase.

As you repeat each phrase, just imagine, visualize, and feel the change happening. By imagining, visualizing, and feeling the direction given in each phrase, you are stating your will in a language your body can understand and cooperate with. You're offering your body direction in a passive way, without using force and without trying to make anything happen.

Quietly let the change happen, using your body's natural tendency to follow your lead. Now, you can start to feel more comfortable. Continue to breathe deeply and slowly and repeat quietly to yourself the following:

I feel quiet. I am beginning to feel quite relaxed—my feet feel quiet and relaxed. My ankles, my knees, and my hips feel light, calm, and comfortable. My stomach and the entire center of my body feel light, calm, and comfortable.

My entire body feels quiet, calm, and comfortable. My arms and my hands feel quiet and warm. My entire body feels quiet and warm. I feel calm and relaxed. My hands feel calm, relaxed, and warm. My hands are relaxed. My hands are warm. My hands are slowly becoming warmer and warmer as I continue to breathe deeply and slowly.

My entire body is quiet, calm, and comfortable. My mind is quiet. I withdraw myself from my surroundings and feel serene and still. My thoughts are turning inward. I feel at ease. Within myself I can visualize and experience myself as quiet, calm, and comfortable. In an easy, quiet, inward-turned way, I am quietly alert. My mind is calm and quiet. I feel an inward quietness.

I will continue with these thoughts for two minutes and then softly open my eyes feeling fine, relaxed, quietly alert, and better than before. It will be interesting to discover how deeply relaxed I can become in a time that normally would seem so short. But even a few minutes of clock time can be all the time in the world for the subconscious mind to dream, to problem-solve, and to achieve deep relaxation and recuperation.

Allow two minutes to pass before you say to yourself or record the last sentence of this exercise that will bring you back to a state of quiet alertness.

You can now slowly open your eyes, stretch, and feel adequately, quietly alert and completely relaxed, comfortable, and better than before.

Regaining Cognitive Control

A few thousand years ago the Stoic philosopher Epictetus wrote the underlying principle of cognitive control, "Man is disturbed not by things, but by the views he takes of them." Four hundred years ago William Shakespeare repeated the concept through his character of Hamlet, "There is nothing either good or bad, but thinking makes it so." Today, we might say that you can learn to *choose how to act* rather than simply react to life events and your own thoughts and emotions.

Your thoughts and reflexes may react somewhat randomly, but you can focus your attention and choose the thoughts, feelings, and behaviors that are most consistent with your current values, skills, and goals.

If, for example, falling rocks hit several people, each would react reflexively to the pain. But their subsequent thoughts and feelings would be determined by their view of themselves, their beliefs about how the world works, and by their ability to exercise cognitive control. One might think, "I'm being hit with rocks. What's wrong with me? I guess I did something bad." Another might think and feel, "I'm not going to let these rocks bother me." And still another might say: "I don't like being hit with rocks. This hurts. I'm getting out of here."

You can develop a variety of helpful thoughts that replace irrational beliefs and debilitating thoughts and reactions. Relaxation, for example, is incompatible with stress and activates a different nervous system. By recognizing debilitating, stress-provoking thoughts and then replacing them with facilitating ones, you can learn to exercise cognitive control and physical control.

A diagnosis of a life-threatening or chronic illness will most likely trigger a reaction of distress or panic in anyone. This is the time to use your cognitive skills to identify those thoughts and feelings that are the most useful to you and to ward off the ones that would only cause more stress.

In his film, *The Healing Force*, the late Norman Cousins, former editor-in-chief of the *Saturday Review*, described his heart attack experience and how he directed the paramedics to turn off the siren and drive at a safe speed. He knew that he would only make things worse if he let himself be caught up in the panic-emergency scenario that usually takes place when someone has a heart attack.

Prior to his own heart attack, Cousins had the opportunity to observe a fellow golfer turn ashen with panic when he had a heart attack and the paramedics hurriedly hooked him up to monitoring devices and began their work. Cousins, recognizing that something had to be done to make human contact with this man and undo his panic, put his hand on the man's shoulder and said, "Sir, you've got a great heart . . . and you're going to be fine. In just a few minutes you'll be in the best hospital in the world." Hearing this, the man lifted his head and opened his eyes. Soon the color came back in his cheeks, and within minutes his heart rate had calmed down.

Five Steps to Integrating Physical and Cognitive Control

An effective way to calm the panic response and soothe your body is to combine relaxation techniques with cognitive control as illustrated in the following exercise. Notice that you are speaking to your body as if talking to a frightened child or animal.

You are the wise, compassionate adult who finally shows up to listen to your mind and body and to protect them from their fears. You'll start with a mental rehearsal that will reveal your initial responses to stressful scenes so you can replace them with self-soothing exercises and thoughts.

Read the exercise through first, or have someone read it to you. Start by sitting upright in a chair with your feet flat on the floor and close your eyes.

1. Mental Rehearsal

Imagine you're calling your doctor or going to receive your treatment and just notice the reactions in your body—changes in heart beat, breathing, and muscle tension. Use your awareness of these stress symptoms to remind yourself to take three slow, deep breaths in three parts: one, inhale; two, hold your breath and tighten the muscles of your stomach, fists, biceps, and legs; and three, exhale slowly and completely as you release muscle tension and float down into the support of the chair and the floor.

2. Notice Any Negative Thoughts

Think of them as old habits that will float away if you don't take them too seriously. They're just thoughts that your worrying mind repeats over and over again. Respond to them with either, "Stop! You're not running my life anymore. I'm here and ready to choose what to do." Or, use the one recommended for developing greater mind-body cooperation:

> Yes, I know your worries better than anyone else. I know where they come from. And, now, I'm taking responsibility for what I choose to do. I won't make you feel bad if something unpleasant happens. You are safe with me.

You might add, "I apologize for not showing up earlier. I'm here now to play my proper leadership role. You are no longer alone."

3. Show Compassion toward the Frightened, Stressed Parts of Yourself

Shift to a protective role in which you—from your strongest, integrated self—speak up and stand up for the more frightened parts of yourself. Your leadership and protective roles empower you to take charge of your life even if smaller, more primitive parts experience fear and self-doubt. You now have a job to do as an active patient.

Your commitment to do the right thing for your body and your life gives you the strength to overcome your fears. As you show up as the leader in your life you tap into the power of an integrated brain—right brain working with left brain hemisphere—and the integration of your conscious mind with your subconscious genius. You now have expanded your identity and resources to be more than your fears and worries.

Continue with three-part breathing and, as you exhale and float down into the chair and floor, acknowledge your connection with the support of the earth and the laws of nature. Acknowledge and feel the support of something much larger, stronger and wiser than your ego struggling as if alone.

4. Make Yourself Safe

Protect your sense of worth from self-criticism and judgment and you'll feel more secure against the threats that cause most of your stress. You are the most distressed when you perceive something or someone as a threat to your self-worth. Once you take your self-worth off the bargaining table, the events of life become simply tasks and challenges that require work, adjustment, and new learning. They no longer are able to threaten your worth and, therefore, can't cause panic or the adrenaline, survival-stress response.

Too many of us learn to gamble with our sense of worth, betting it on getting a good grade in school or on being popular or achieving our goals. It's as if we're telling ourselves, "If it's sunny outside, I'll feel good. If it rains, I'll feel bad. If she likes me, I'll feel good. If she doesn't like me, I'll feel bad." It's rather like that childhood game of picking the petals off a daisy so it can tell us, "She loves me; she loves me not." You take something as innate and valuable as your self-worth and put it up to be judged and determined by events and people outside your control, thereby, making yourself vulnerable to stress.

This aspect of stress management training is based on maintaining a deep, inner sense of safety that comes from knowing that your self-respect and self-worth are secure against anything that happens out there. Regardless of what happens or what anyone says, your worth is safe.

Practice using your three-part breathing technique to communicate, "It's safe to exhale. It's safe to let go of muscle tension. Your worth is safe with me. I am choosing to be here and face this task." With these messages of safety, your body will soon learn to stop the stress hormones in less than thirty seconds. See a longer list of messages of safety in appendix B, "Reducing Stress by Making Yourself Safe with You," and read them to yourself every day.

Sure, it's good to feel happy when things are going well, but real confidence means knowing that, even when things aren't going well, you can minimize the pain in your life, maximize the joy, and get on with your life as best you can.

5. Accept Yourself As Human

Having a solid sense of self-worth doesn't mean that you think you're better than anyone else or that you're perfect. It means that you acknowledge your human imperfections without shame and accept yourself as being *perfectly* human.

Accepting your humanity also means that you stand up for your feelings regardless of what anyone says or thinks. You don't have to be defensive about any aspect of yourself that others may criticize. You no longer have to try to be perfect in a fruitless attempt to avoid mistakes or criticism. Your worth is solid, and, therefore, you can accept helpful feedback on how to improve, but you don't have to tolerate abusive attacks.

As you practice these concepts and principles of an innate worth that is not available for judgment, your feelings of safety will follow, and your stress levels will decrease. Soon, the look in your eyes and everything about you will communicate:

- I have worth. Regardless of my condition, I have a right to be here.

- I don't need to apologize to anyone for my existence, my human vulnerabilities, or my feelings.

Exercise: Rate Your Stress Level

For one week, rate your stress level on a scale of zero to ten where zero represents when you felt completely safe and ten represents those times when you felt the most stressed. Grade your stress level on a scale of zero to ten.

Safest   *Most Stressed*

0 __ 1 __ 2 __ 3 __ 4 __ 5 __ 6 __ 7 __ 8 __ 9 __ 10 __

Note that you can't have a stress level of ten every day. When you calculate the level of danger, decide if it is close to a ten—a message of extreme danger requiring high levels of adrenaline—or closer to a three, a message of mild disruption. If your earthquake is in this lower range, exhale and think or say, "It's only a three; we're safe. This is not the end of the world for us. Your worth is safe with me." Or "I will not let this ruin our weekend or our evening."

By gauging your level of stress every day for one week, you'll discover that not every stressful event has to be an "end of the world" level-ten disaster. You'll be amazed to discover that your body and (autonomic nervous system?) will follow your message of safety, quickly lower your heart rate and stress hormones, and allow you to be effective and productive in less than a minute.

- I can maintain my self-respect and self-worth regardless of life's problems and tasks.

As every part of you learns that you will stand up for yourself and put a limit to self-induced stress, you'll find that there's very little that can evoke a stress response for more than a few moments. After all, your worth and your body are safe with you. You don't need a stress-survival response except for those rare occasions when you need to run from or fight a physical threat. You now give yourself a psychological and emotional safety net of unassailable self-worth that will catch you whenever you fall and will hold you.

This chapter has presented you with several important concepts and techniques. However, don't let the techniques distract you away from the main point. You can facilitate your body's coping mechanisms by learning how to minimize stress and worry. When you combine physical and cognitive coping strategies, you have powerful tools for reducing stress and focusing your body's energies on recuperation and repair.

Chapter 5

Coping with Depression and Helplessness

It is not until mature individuals see that they are the creator of their own Self that the search of an external paradise gives way to self-soothing and internal sense of bliss.

— Joseph Campbell, *The Power of Myth*

When the diagnosis is cancer, you can expect feelings of depression, with its symptoms of irritability, fatigue, hopelessness, and insomnia. At times the only healthy reaction is to be depressed, at least temporarily. After all, loss of health and possibly your former lifestyle caused by illness is an occasion for sadness and mourning, if not deep, temporary depression. In fact, it may be healthier to acknowledge that you feel depressed and express your feelings now rather than trying to suppress them and risk chronic depression later.

While many consider depression to be a "negative emotion," it is in fact one natural mechanism for coping with shock by conserving energy and providing time to think about ways of adjusting to traumatic change.

Cancer and Depression

In general, cancer patients are no more depressed than patients with other physical illnesses. New York's Memorial Sloan-Kettering Cancer Center has determined that the percentage of cancer patients with significant depression is similar to the percentage among patients seriously ill with other diseases—between 20 and 25 percent. Yet cancer patients tend to be given less antidepressant medication than other patients because it is assumed that having cancer must be depressing. If you experience symptoms of depression and anxiety, therefore, you may need to insist that you receive supportive counseling and, if necessary, medication.

The Psychiatry Service of Memorial Sloan-Kettering reports that half of the cancer patients they see have suffered from acute stress and "reactive," as opposed to "chronic" psychological depression. Patients can more easily handle the relatively short-term, reactive depression that often accompanies the stress of a cancer diagnosis if they allow themselves a period of mourning or grieving. Put simply, you can manage and recover from your depression if you acknowledge your loss—loss of control, loss of part of your body, and loss of your self-image or identity as a healthy person who thought of yourself as invulnerable to illness.

For the large majority of cancer patients, the depressive reaction could subside within a few weeks, but additional periods of depression may occur at various stages of the cancer experience and in response to changes in cancer therapy. You can manage these transient forms of depression with professional and family support, active involvement in treatment, and by maintaining some control over your treatment and environment.

Options for Therapy and Medication

With the more serious forms of depression—found more frequently in older patients with advanced stages of cancer—symptoms continue for longer than a few weeks and may involve an overwhelming sense of being a burden to loved ones and feelings of hopelessness. While suicide among cancer patients is rare, suicidal thoughts may increase. This doesn't mean a patient wants to die, even if he or she says so, but rather that they wish to end their physical discomfort and loss of their former activities. In such cases, give serious consideration to seeking psychotherapy, and possibly medication. You don't have to suffer alone with the painful hurt of depression.

Physical Depression

While depression is usually thought of as being emotional, it also can be physical when your body turns its resources inward to cope with healing and recovery. In fact, shock, coma, sleep, and depression may all be very similar states in which the brain directs energy away from external activity toward rapid healing. It is also possible that with trauma, the brain needs time and energy to dream while it searches its vast resources for a solution.

Many of the symptoms of depression—feeling sad, guilty, overburdened, irritable, and withdrawn—can be caused by physical illness or by the side effects of cancer therapy. Decreased levels of activity, difficulty relating, insomnia, loss of appetite, fatigue, headaches, and loss of sexual interest can be signs of both a physical as well as a psychological-emotional depression. Depressive symptoms can be aggravated by drugs (for example, Compazine and drugs that suppress your hormones) or can be the result of pancreatic cancer or brain tumors. Do not, therefore, allow anyone—including your doctor—to tell you that your symptoms are "just an emotional response."

Three Contributors to Depression

1. Expectations of Control

Life-threatening disasters and illnesses disrupt your illusion of control and order. Cancer throws all your plans and schedules into an upheaval. The more you try to hold onto your need for control, the greater will be your sense of loss of control and your vulnerability to depression.

Our modern society creates the expectation that we can get what we want when we want it. It also creates a fear of loss of control if events don't fit neatly with our schedule and expectations. Jet planes and motorboats take us around the globe and against the wind and tide, distorting the mind's sense of time and distance to such an extent that our bodies suffer jet lag while trying to adapt to the rapid change.

Modern "advances" reinforce an illusion of control and lead us to believe that we can assert our wills on the earth with our bulldozers, on animal life with our chemicals, on peoples with our weapons, and on our own bodies with drugs and medical technology. Our culture has lost touch with the native peoples' reverence for the Earth and the wisdom of working with, instead of against, nature.

In today's world, you can use a motor boat to cut through the waves in a direct line to your destination, oblivious of the tides and winds. But to operate a sailboat you must learn to appreciate the power of the wind and the sea and be willing to work in humble accord with them. In the world of the sailboat, however, points of destination and times of arrival can only be approximations—the expression of a wish, never a demand. At sea, it would be fool-hardy to act as if you could totally control or ignore nature.

In sailing, as in life, you must steer around obstacles, take into account unpredictable changes in the environment, and learn to use the current to your advantage. To reach your destination you must approach it in a series of turns ("tacks") that seem to take you away from your goal. You cannot sail directly into the wind toward your goal. From the modern perspective the need to reassess goals and change direction is often misinterpreted as a failure and a cause for upset that life is not conforming to our schedule. In fact, a willingness to adjust to an ever-changing reality is a rational act of humility that helps reduce stress, frustration, and depression.

2. Learned Helplessness

Hospitalization tends to regress most patients—even when they are doctors—to the early childhood experience of dependency. This regression is called "learned helplessness." To combat this form of depression you may need to revive a sense of being effective and see a connection between your actions and results.

Children—whether raised in a ghetto or in a mansion—who are taught that what they do has little effect on what happens to them will develop a passive, helpless attitude toward life. In contrast, children who discover that they can be effective in learning new skills, reaching their goals, and receiving rewards, will develop a sense of resilience to subsequent challenges. Supported by their early victories they can survive the most bitter deprivation and punishment to become physically and mentally healthy and socially successful.

It is essential, therefore, that patients learn that they can have some control over their medical treatment, meals, hospital conditions, and life decisions. When you can't get what you want and do what you want in so many areas of your life, it becomes imperative that you become effective in managing your attitude and emotional states.

The pressure to conform to a passive-patient role is so strong in many hospitals that you may need the support of your family and friends to overcome this form of learned helplessness and the feelings of depression that go with it.

3. A Refusal to Mourn

Depression has been defined as "a refusal to mourn." That is, depression—and, I would include frustration and struggle—may be caused or maintained by refusing to acknowledge your losses and insisting that you should be in control. It is difficult to admit that, as a human being, your control over life events is limited and that you may not be able to prevent the loss of your own health or that of your loved ones.

Refusing to mourn the loss of this illusion of infinite powers often shows itself in the form of persistent thoughts such as:

- Why did it happen?

- What did I do wrong?

- What should I have done to prevent it?

- What's wrong with me?

The focus of these thoughts is on the past and the fantasy that you could or should have been able to prevent the painful event. It also seems to serve the purpose of avoiding confrontation with something deeper and, perhaps, more painful, the fact that you are not all-powerful; you cannot control everything; and that, like all humans, you are vulnerable to illness and death. Refusing to accept these facts of life can keep you stuck in a battle against reality and in anger at yourself for being human. In essence, this is a refusal to accept yourself as human—in some ways very powerful and in other ways limited. Once you start to accept yourself as human, appropriate feelings of sadness and grief will replace depression, struggle, frustration, and anger.

How to Cope with Depression: Four Steps

1. Acknowledge the Limits of Control

The first step out of depression is to acknowledge that you have limited control over life, so you stop beating yourself up for what happened. Then, you can focus your energy on taking charge of what is under your control, your attitude and your ability to feel compassion for all those who suffer. Even if every other aspect of your life is out of your control, you always can take some control over how you treat yourself. Acknowledging limited control doesn't mean you're giving up. It means you're focusing your energies on what you can control.

By accepting your human vulnerabilities and limits, you can minimize self-blame and self-criticism, forgive yourself for being human, and have compassion for all humans, including yourself. The ironic thing about control is that the more you try to get it, the more frustrated, inadequate, and out-of-control you will feel. The more you acknowledge the limits of your control, the more you can focus on what is under your control, thereby increasing your effectiveness. The theologian Reinhold Niebuhr has encapsulated this concept in a brief prayer altered slightly by Alcoholics Anonymous:

> Grant me the serenity
> To accept the things I cannot change;
> Courage to change the things I can;
> And wisdom to know the difference.

You can gain inner peace and stress reduction by relaxing your attempt to change other people, the weather, or the inevitability of death and taxes. Accept that many events in life will be just different from what you prefer and expect and yet not be "bad." Relax your expectation that things should be your way, and you will find that life holds many pleasant discoveries and surprises.

A fellow psychologist told me of an experience he had that illustrates this point:

> One morning I started my day, as usual, by making orange juice from frozen concentrate. I mixed the juice, poured myself a glass, and tasted it. "It's bad! It's spoiled," I said to myself as I began to pour the remainder down the drain. Then I paused and thought that in the hundreds of times that I had made orange juice I had never encountered juice that had spoiled. "How can that be?" So I retrieved the empty can for a closer look. On re-examination I read the label and discovered that I had mistakenly bought a can of tangerine juice. Tasting the juice again, I realized that it wasn't spoiled or bad; it was just different—different from what I had expected.

The first step out of chronic depression is to accept that just because things are out of your control and don't go the way you expected, they are not necessarily bad and awful. Accepting that, as a human being, you do not have god-like control over life is the first step toward realistic control, productive activity, and resourceful coping with depression and cancer.

2. *Choose What You Will Do*

Most of the time we humans live by the principle of "seek pleasure and avoid pain." But, fortunately our higher brain grants us the ability to delay pleasure and choose to face pain for a "higher," long-term good. You can choose to face a difficult task now, like getting a root canal, to avoid greater pain in the future. You can even overcome your natural tendency to avoid pain by imagining the benefits of undergoing surgery and taking chemotherapy in order to prolong your life. No other creature has the human ability to choose pain and difficulty to achieve a higher good in the future.

The second step out of depression is to use your human ability to choose what to do for the long-term benefit of your body and your life. By choosing what to do you break free of the inner conflict between the part of you that says, "You have to do this difficult, painful thing." and the part that says, "I don't want to."

Of course you don't *want* to face surgery, pain, chemotherapy, hair loss, and nausea. You don't have to *want to* do these difficult things and you certainly shouldn't wait until you want to do them. Nor is it helpful to tell yourself, "You *have to* do something awful that you're not going to want to do. But you have to because you're a victim."

This ineffective inner dialogue—repeated dozens of times a day—contributes to depression, resistance, foot-dragging, resentment, and loss of motivation as you try to make yourself do something that you have not fully chosen.

Observe your reactions when you tell yourself you have to do something. You're telling yourself that you're being controlled by others who are making you do something you don't want to do. You're hypnotizing yourself into feeling like a victim and you're denying your unique human ability to make choices—even tough choices.

You can stop confusing your mind and body by saying, "If I'm going to do it, I will fully choose and commit to it. If I choose not do it or choose to delay doing it, I will accept the consequences. I'm in charge of my life."

I choose is not just a phrase, it's a leadership act that shifts your brain and body to mobilize your energy and direct it toward making your treatment easier, less painful, and less depressing.

3. Define the Problem as Something You Can Work on Now

Are you defining your problem or task as coping with and surviving cancer or trying to change the past? When you define your problem as "I have cancer" or "something awful happened to me twenty years ago," you're creating frustration for your body because it can't release its energy to work in the past. Being diagnosed with cancer *was* a traumatic event that will require some period of grieving, but it is not a problem with which you can struggle today. It's a challenging fact that happened in the past. You can only work in the present—the only time in which you can be effective—to deal with that fact and to live to your fullest, each moment.

If you hear yourself saying, "I'm depressed because I have cancer," you might respond, "I'm so sorry. Of course I feel depressed. That's awful." But you can't help yourself move out of depression until you stop seeing your problem as something that happened to you in the past.

You might encourage a shift to what you can do now that this awful thing has happened by saying to yourself, "I have every right to cry and to take time to grieve and feel depressed. When I've processed these feelings, I'll start a plan to do what I can to improve the quality of my life and my chances of survival."

4. Take One More Step

When you're in the midst of depression, it's easy to feel overwhelmed by all you have to do medically, emotionally, and for the family. You can't possibly do the infinite number of tasks that require your full attention, and you simply do not have available the enormous levels of energy required. You don't know where to start, and you feel as if you'll fail miserably at whatever you do. So it's too easy to lose sight of what's right in front of you that you can start working on now.

When I completed chemotherapy in December 1975, I was exhausted, bald, and beardless, and had lost most of my eyebrows and eyelashes. By June 1976, most of my hair and beard had returned, and I had the energy to take my first trip to Europe for seven weeks. The next year I visited the famous hypnotist Dr. Milton H. Erickson and asked him, "What can I tell cancer patients?" As was his style, Dr. Erickson, who seldom gave a direct answer, responded with this story.

> A number of years ago a story of a terrible tragedy appeared in the newspaper. It was sunset on Lake Michigan when a storm quickly came up, surprising a sailing party, and capsizing their boat thirteen miles from shore. The passengers quickly panicked. Some were so overwhelmed by the enormity of the task of swimming thirteen miles, they never even tried. Others vigorously attempted to reach shore but rapidly exhausted themselves. Some must have cursed themselves for their mistakes, for having taken the cruise, or for being unprepared for the storm. They spent their last moments in self-blame and regrets.
>
> There was only one survivor, a young girl. No one knows how she avoided or overcame the panic of all those around her, and, no doubt, her own panic, but

they found her the next morning on the shore. She was moving her arms in the sand, repeating to herself over and over again, "I can swim one stroke more. I can swim one stroke more."

That's how you complete any enormous, overwhelming task of survival. You don't have to feel confident or know that you can do it, but you start doing whatever you can do, You take one more stroke, one more step.

Regardless of the size of your task or goal, you cannot finish it all at once; you can only begin the journey now. Finishing and achieving are in the future, beyond your control. All you can do—all you ever have to do—is to choose to start now for five, fifteen, or thirty minutes to take one more step toward nourishing and exercising your body, toward facing another round of medical therapies. You only need to deal with this moment—that's all there ever is.

Just facing the day can be too large a task when your energy is low and your hopes are even lower. Facing cancer and all your questions about the meaning of cancer is too large a task to tackle all at once. It's quite enough to just get yourself out of bed by literally taking that first step to get your feet on the floor. You then find the energy to take one more step, then another to wash, eat, walk, telephone, write, or whatever you choose to face. You'll have broken free of inertia and discover an unstoppable momentum that allows you to move forward, to savor small pleasures in your day, and awaken a life force that wants to live your unique version of life.

Chapter 6

Becoming an Active Patient

Fighting cancer involves more than excising a tumor and focusing our latest weapons on the metastases. It must include recognition by both the medical profession and the patient, that the patient's mind and body are powerful factors in this fight. Effective cancer therapy includes treating the healthy portion of your body and psyche as well as combating the diseased cells.

You Are More Than Your Diagnosis

You are more than the host of a serious illness. You have a mind and feelings and a body that is largely healthy. Failure to use these resources and to recognize what you have to contribute to the battle against cancer can lead to passivity, resistance, stress, and difficulty completing life-saving treatments.

When doctors affirm a faith in your body's own healing power and a respect for you as a whole person, they are performing at their very best. Good doctors want to do everything they can to save your life. Yet technological advances and the tendency toward specialization increase the danger of treating you simply as an interesting diagnosis or the site for a battle between modern science and death. From this bias, the natural fighting potential of your body and the essential contribution you make by expressing your emotions and thoughts are often overlooked or minimized.

While you may not be an expert with regard to cancer therapy, you do know that you'll need time to adjust to the medical procedures, to surgery, and to the side effects of cancer therapy. You can achieve this adjustment more easily when you consciously choose your treatment based on knowledge of your needs, what the doctors have told you, and in consideration of the kind of life you wish to live after cancer therapy.

The Patient Role: Mastery or Helplessness

Being diagnosed with a life-threatening illness often creates a wish to be taken care of by the experts. When you're sick, you have permission to let go of your daily pressures and obligations while your body takes time to heal and your mind takes time to adjust to the changes that illness can bring to your life.

Ironically, as you let go of one set of responsibilities from your usual roles, you assume another series of obligations and shoulds from your patient role. Pressure from doctors, from the hospital staff, and from your family can add a new sense of burden and, with cancer especially, deeper feelings of helplessness.

Because of the highly specialized knowledge required to make an accurate cancer diagnosis and an effective treatment plan, cancer patients are especially prone to feeling helpless and passive. Your own wish to depend on the expertise of others, therefore, combined with the rules and routines of the hospital and the complexity of cancer therapy constellate to diminish your usual sense of being in charge of your life.

The passivity of the typical patient role and the rigidity of the hospital environment promote the feeling that your efforts are futile. While hospital efficiency may be promoted by control over how the patient dresses, their visiting hours, and when he wakes up, it does not promote health. Being stripped of control over the simple, but individual, choices in your day can lead to depression.

My Heart Attacked Me—My Cells Have Turned Against Me

Patients with life-threatening illnesses such as cancer and heart disease tend to feel helpless in controlling their own bodies. It can seem as if your very cells have gone crazy and, as one patient said, "my heart attacked me." It is essential for your psychological wellbeing, therefore, that you learn ways of calming your body and becoming active in taking as much control as you would like over your hospital environment and treatment.

Becoming an active patient is not only good for your emotional wellbeing, it may also improve your chances of survival. A study at the University of California, San Francisco, involving patients with melanoma found that active participation was associated with significantly smaller tumors and significantly more white cells at the site of the tumor.

One of the major adaptive tasks confronting the seriously ill is maintaining a sense of competence and mastery. In order to do this you must alter your expectations regarding what you can do for yourself and what requires the assistance of others. While you shouldn't expect to feel a sense of mastery overnight, you can start by redefining the patient or sick role so that it fits your needs and not just those of the doctor and the hospital.

One patient's response to the patient's role was poignantly reported by his wife, in their book, *Heartsounds*. Dr. Hal Lear was an urologist who had treated many patients with serious illnesses, including cancer. Now he was a patient himself, with heart disease, and like his own patients he had to struggle with his reactions to his doctors and his new role, finally coming to this insight:

> I know they want to help me. But I also know they can be fallible, and they are busy. I've been too passively accepting the patient's role ... they give no credence to my description of my condition. They are missing the boat again. And I want to have more control at the helm of this boat.

Becoming an Effective Human Being

In May 1982, a consortium of health care facilities in the San Francisco Bay Area brought together physicians, nurses, hospital administrators, scholars from the humanities, and patients to consider what factors constitute an "effective health care decision." The participants in this consortium acknowledged that too often hospitalization and medical treatment severely impair the patient's self-image, ability to function with dignity, and sense of effectiveness. They concluded that while the longevity of the patient, cost-benefit considerations, and social impact were important criteria, patient participation in, and patient satisfaction with, the decision-making process were the paramount determinants of an effective health care decision.

Strong support for patient participation in treatment decisions, for actively seeking information about illness and health issues, and for expressing negative emotions, is mounting from the research on improved chances of survival and adaptation to illness. No longer will the quiet, passive, compliant patient be looked upon as virtuous and the vocal, questioning patient as a nuisance.

In summary, they echoed the sentiments of Professor Martin Seligman, former president of the American Psychological Association, "The central goal in successful therapy should be to have the patient come to believe that his responses produce the gratification he desires—that he is, in short, an effective human being."

Being a Good Patient May Not Be Good for You

Trying to be a pleasant, "good patient" who doesn't cause any problems for the medical staff takes a great deal of energy that may be a waste of energy! Because research now suggests that expressing your so-called negative emotions may actually help you to survive longer.

In a Johns Hopkins study of patients with metastatic breast cancer, those patients who, were judged by their doctors to be poorly adjusted to their disease and to have negative attitudes toward their doctors survived longer than another group who expressed positive emotions and attitudes toward their doctors and were judged to be well-adjusted to their illness. Even so, doctors had given the first group a negative prognosis because they had expressed their feelings of depression, anxiety, and alienation.

(Readers should note that women with localized breast cancer now have a very good chance of surviving their disease. The women in this study had cancer that had spread beyond the original site, and if they were treated today, would have a much greater chance of survival and cure.)

These findings do *not* suggest that you should try to change how you feel. Each of us has our own schedule for releasing emotion. The main point to be gathered from this research is that you can stop trying to be a good patient, and you can stop trying to hold back so-called negative emotions. And you can watch for the day when the so-called bad patients with the negative emotions will be the ones considered well-adjusted to their disease and as having a better prognosis.

Who Knows What's Best for You?

As you become a more active patient, you'll learn that you and your doctor will sometimes have different ideas about what you need to do medically. Doctors are trained to fight diseases and to save lives. From their point of view, often the "most aggressive" or "radical" surgical procedures make sense. Dr. Keith W. Sehnert, in *How to Be Your Own Doctor—Sometimes*, writes that too many patients don't question, challenge, or doubt their doctors. He recounts a yarn about a woman who telephoned her doctor asking him to examine her long-invalided husband, Henry, who had, she said, "taken a turn for the worse."

> The doctor got to her home as fast as he could, but by the time he arrived Henry showed no sign of breathing. Being unable to find a pulse, the doctor sadly told the

new widow that her husband was dead. Upon hearing this Henry bolted upright in his bed and proclaimed, "I am not!" His wife immediately pushed him back onto the pillow and ordered, "Now lie down, Henry; the doctor knows best!"

Too many patients play the patient role to the extreme, accepting the doctor's opinion and the medical perspective without question. Later they worry about unanswered questions or the side effects of a medication, but are fearful of calling the busy doctor. According to Dr. Sehnert, "the activated patient doesn't leave the doctor's office saying: 'Gosh, what a doctor! He didn't explain anything to me.' The activated patient asks questions—lots of them. If he doesn't get answers, or even worse, is put down, the activated patient considers finding another doctor."

Know Your Doctor's Assumptions

Doctors tend to assume that you are in agreement with them or that you are leaving all decisions to them. If you are comfortable with this approach and with the results of the procedures recommended by your doctor, you will probably adapt to your illness as well as anyone who chooses to discuss alternatives with his doctor.

If, however, you have doubts about the recommended procedure, or about your ability to live with the possible results, you need to make this clear. Don't assume—like Henry's wife—that the doctor knows what's best for you!

Even if you agree with the necessity of radical surgery, you need to inform your doctor of whether or not reconstruction or prosthetics is important to you. As with the example of breast surgery, the patient's wishes for breast reconstruction may only be possible if discussed with the surgeon and a plastic surgeon beforehand. Men undergoing certain forms of chemotherapy or radiation that damage sperm cells should be provided with information about sperm banks but sometimes are not. Both men and women who want to have children in the future need to tell their doctors. Remember: Doctors tend to be focused on saving you from cancer. Fighting for the quality of your life after cancer is primarily your concern and your responsibility. It's important enough to be stated again: Regardless of your type of cancer or medical procedure, don't assume that your doctor knows what you want and need!

This is not the time to be timid. Let your doctor know what you are expecting and ask questions about any worries you have. Let him or her know if you want a partnership based on frank and open dialogue.

With the urgency that surrounds cancer treatment, little time is typically taken to discuss your emotional and lifestyle needs. Let your doctor know what side effects you're willing to live with and which ones seem to be an unnecessary impairment of the quality of your life with little apparent improvement in your overall chances for survival. Discuss with your doctor any fears you may have about potential side effects, any thoughts about alternative treatments, and any wishes for a second opinion.

Get help in clarifying your feelings and presenting your ideas. Keep in mind that you can benefit from patient support groups, psychotherapists, and the support of your family and friends. Feel free to fill the doctor's office with advisors, advocates, family members, and friends. There's strength in numbers!

Most doctors will welcome a patient who, through seeking a second opinion, asking questions, and reading, freely and consciously chooses both the doctor and the procedures recommended. Those physicians who are worried about the authority of their roles will refuse to have dialogues with their patients and will only work with patients who remain passive and childlike.

The rationale frequently offered for this approach to the doctor-patient relationship is that patients want to be passive and that they are often in a regressed, childlike state. When we consider the emotional impact of cancer, it becomes evident that temporary passivity is to be expected in any person who faces a catastrophic illness. And the diagnosis of cancer is enough to shock anyone into a passive and dependent state. But it should not be assumed that this will be a permanent condition. Just as you are more than your disease, you are more than your temporary helplessness and dependency. A balance between activity and passivity and independence and dependence will be more readily achieved as patients assume, and are allowed to assume, their proper role of participation and control. If you are more comfortable with a less active approach and with the procedures recommended by your doctor, you'll probably adapt to your illness as well as anyone who chooses to discuss alternatives with his or her doctor.

The Power of Choice

A sense of mastery and control over your life as a cancer patient can begin with some influence over your surroundings, such as choice of room furnishings and meals, and participation in decisions about the timing of medical procedures. This level of control, if given to all patients, would help minimize the passivity and infantilizing aspects of the "sick role."

Today, many patients use the Internet to actively participate in their healthcare decisions by accessing information about their disease, treatment options, and the latest clinical trials for their disease. (For information on clinical trails, see the National Cancer Institute's website at www.nci.nih.gov/clinicaltrials.)

In order to make an informed choice and to give informed consent to your cancer therapy, you may want information about your disease, treatment alternatives, and side effects. While you might fear becoming pessimistic if you learn too much about your cancer, research has shown that becoming well-informed actually helps sustain hopeful attitudes. Having the facts, for most patients, helps to overcome the anxiety associated with uncertainty and unrealistic fears.

Though today's patients seem to prefer more detailed information about their cancer, not all patients feel this way. In a University of Pennsylvania Cancer Center study, an average of 6 to 7 percent of patients indicated that they did not want specific items of information. So, while most patients want more information, preferences vary, depending on the type of information, the age and culture of the patient, and the patient's individual needs.

The preference for more information and participation is highest among younger patients who were raised in a culture that is less trusting of authority and one in which medical information is readily available to the layman. Older patients, in general, tend to hold to the old adage that "doctor knows best."

Health care providers ought to take these individual preferences into consideration when offering information. They could give patients an opportunity to exercise freedom of choice and to avoid unnecessary anxiety by simply asking, "Do you have any questions about your illness and treatment plan?" or "would you like more detailed information about alternative treatments?"

It's natural to want to know about, and to control, what's happening to you. When patients are denied information and their control over their lives is limited, they are more likely to turn to unconventional therapies or to noncompliance as ways of exercising control.

In an attempt to discover why so many cancer patients turn to unproven or unconventional treatments, Dr. Neil Ellison began a nationwide search for patients who tried unconventional or metabolic therapies such as laetrile, diets, vitamin therapy, and chelation agents. (Chelation is a controversial and unproven procedure in which a synthetic amino acid is used to bind with calcium and minerals in the bloodstream that are then excreted from the body.) In this National Cancer Institute study, it was found that a majority of the patients who had turned to these treatments had been told by their physicians, directly or through their families, that they had a "terminal disease and that nothing else can be done." This pronouncement by their doctors left the patients feeling abandoned and hopeless. This situation resulted in what Dr. Ellison called,

... blind dependence on any treatment offering cure, palliation, or the faintest glimmer of optimism ... Metabolic therapy intimately involves the patient in the day-to-day treatment of his disease. Almost all patients were required to alter their life-styles and were thus constantly reminded of this involvement. They did more than simply make an appointment for chemotherapy. This ability to control or influence one's own treatment must be of tremendous psychologic importance . . . the patient must be made *more involved in therapeutic decisions and disease treatments.* Perhaps if these goals are accomplished, many well-intended but misguided patients will not turn to quackery or charlatans for care. [Emphasis added.]

For patients who are in a delicate state of health, every bit of control over their bodies and surroundings can mean a return to feelings of power and purpose. As more patients become active and informed consumers of healthcare services, doctors and nurses will become more patient-centered and start to include patients in the decision-making process. Doctors will begin sharing the information and authority necessary for patients to become active members of the health care team. Playing a more active role will not only boost the spirits of patients, it may also improve their chances of surviving life-threatening illness.

Chapter 7

You and Your Doctor—Building a Working Relationship

When choosing a doctor with whom you can build a collaborative relationship for your health, you may want to apply your comparison-shopping skills to find a doctor who has experience with your illness, treats you with respect, and includes you as part of the treatment team.

Unfortunately, a warm bedside manner and technical expertise don't always come in the same individual. That's another reason you'll want to create a team that includes those who can offer emotional and psychological support—perhaps your family doctor, a medical social worker, therapist or chaplain, and family and friends.

How to Find a Quality Doctor and a First-Rate Hospital

In her January 5, 2009 *New York Times* health column, Denise Grady tells of a relative diagnosed with rectal cancer who avoided the need for a colostomy bag because she found a surgeon who specializes in rectal cancer rather than following the advice of a surgeon at her nearby community hospital. Grady writes that the two-hour trip to get a second opinion at a teaching hospital was "worth the trouble."

Combining mutual respect and competent care in the doctor-patient relationship is possible, but may require exerting some effort. In your search for the right kind of doctor for you, it may be useful to follow one or more of the following suggestions:

- Ask a nurse, "Who's the best doctor in this department (e.g., in the oncology, gastroenterology, gynecology, or urology departments)?" Be specific about the type of doctor-patient relationship you're looking for.

- Ask patients with a similar diagnosis if they are pleased with their doctor.

- Get a second opinion for any major operation when time permits.

- Look online (www.hospitalcompare.hhs.gov) to find out which hospitals achieve the best results with your illness or surgery. Look for a hospital and doctors that specialize in treating your illness. Those hospitals with 200 or more operations per year of a specific type (for example, open-heart surgery) have 25 to 40 percent lower mortality rates than hospitals doing fewer.

- Check with your county medical society to obtain the names of at least three doctors and their credentials. You can also obtain the names of physicians doing cancer research from the Office of Cancer Communication by phone (301/451-6879), or email (ncioce@mail.nih. gov), or by visiting their website (www.cancer.gov/ aboutnci/oce/page3).

- Consider a teaching hospital if your problem is unusual or if it requires complex treatment. Teaching hospitals tend to be familiar with the latest procedures. If, however, you can get appropriate treatment from your nearby community hospital, it is likely to provide more personal attention and privacy.

- Choose a doctor who treats you as a complete human being with social and financial concerns, beliefs, and emotions.

Understanding the Basic Doctor-Patient Contract

To build a healthy partnership with their doctors, patients need to be aware of their own assumptions and expectations about the doctor-patient relationship. In *The Clay Pedestal*, renowned cardiologist Dr. Thomas Preston writes that within the "basic contract," society grants physicians the exclusive power to be healers and to have dominance over the patient who, in this relationship, is inferior, passive, and very dependent. In the tradition of that outdated basic contract, physicians would assume that their superior knowledge and experience enabled them to judge what information patients should receive and what decisions patients are capable of making. Under this contract, it was standard practice to deny patients the data and alternatives they needed to make an informed decision.

Dr. Preston reminds us that while professional expertise in making medical decisions is indispensable, withholding pertinent information cheats patients of the opportunity to participate in their own healthcare decisions. The best interests of patients are served when patients, not the doctors, decide what they wish to know.

Failure to inform patients of their rights to adjunctive or alternative cancer treatments has been so widespread that in California, doctors are now subject to malpractice suits if they don't give a pamphlet describing the alternatives available to breast cancer patients. This may seem like a sad commentary on the state of the doctor-patient relationship and patient trust, but it highlights the fact that patients and doctors often have very different perspectives and that doctor-patient communications need to be improved.

Realistic Trust or Blind Faith?

Some doctors naturally inspire trust, as did the doctor that treated my mother for uterine cancer. My mother explained how he calmed her fears and won her confidence:

> He listens. He doesn't hover over you, but sits down and doesn't make you feel rushed. He comes in every day,

even after surgery, to see how I'm doing. He explained everything that would happen and introduced me to the rest of the staff. And he's well-liked by the nurses and the staff. They all think highly of him. When I asked about possible pain, he said that he would give me something if I needed it. I knew that he would do his best.

Such basic but essential elements of human contact and sensitivity assured my mother that the doctor respected her needs and feelings and that everything humanly possible would be done to keep her informed and comfortable. Andrew Silk, a young writer with lung cancer, felt he could trust his doctor because of her willingness to share the facts of his condition and her sensitivity to his fears, describing the relationship in this way:

> I was able to cede the responsibility for my treatment to Dr. Moore. She combined quiet authority with careful monitoring and precise reporting of my condition. This alone would not have won her my complete trust. I felt that she was as concerned with ridding me of my belief that I could not be cured as she was with ridding me of the tumor itself. Without her compassionate understanding of my fears, I doubt that I would have allowed her quiet confidence to win me over.

Not every patient has a doctor who takes the time to learn about the patient's beliefs, emotions, and fears. But someone needs to acknowledge the importance of your mind, body, and emotions in your battle against cancer. If your doctor tells you, "your fears are just in your head," or "you should just get over your emotions," you may want to find a doctor who can listen to you, reduce your fears, and thereby help improve your chances of recovery.

In his bestselling book, *Blink,* Malcolm Gladwell, cites the work of medical malpractice lawyer Alice Burkin and medical researcher Wendy Levinson stating, "the risk of being sued for malpractice has very little to do with how many mistakes a doctor makes." This is something that doctors today need to hear. The fact is, patients don't sue doctors they like, and that it's the doctor's tone of voice, not his or her credentials or number of mistakes that determines the likelihood of being sued. Those doctors who sound dominant or superior tend to be sued more often than those who are respectful and listen to their patients. In one study, doctors who spent three minutes longer (on average a total of 18.3 minutes) with each patient had never been sued compared to those who spent only 15 minutes and had been sued.

The authority of a physician can't go unquestioned and the unilateral decisions of a physician can never be accepted with blind faith. In their book, *Your Body, Your Health*, three physicians, Drs. Sobczyk, Shulman, and Fonda encourage patients to stop blindly taking doctor's advice. They remind patients that it is, after all, your body and your life, not your doctor's.

Shared Responsibility, Shared Authority

Some doctors will claim, as mine did, that they are responsible for your life. When I've challenged doctors on this point they told me, "I was taught in medical school that the doctor is the captain of the ship. If a nurse drops a scalpel in the operating room, the doctor is responsible. Medical decisions can't be made by committee."

This argument is often used to convince patients that they have negligible authority and, therefore, little responsibility in the medical setting. Without authority patients are left with only veto power and noncompliance as ways of expressing their opinions and preferences.

Not only is this an unworkable doctor-patient relationship, but it is based on a faulty argument and a faulty definition of responsibility. Some doctors argue that their legal responsibility, which holds them liable for malpractice, supersedes any responsibility patients may have for themselves and for their medical treatment. But legal responsibility is only one type of responsibility.

As the patient—the recipient of medical treatment—you are the one who will live with the outcome. You, therefore, have an essential role and stake in medical decisions. You also are the only one who knows your wishes and values, and you are the one who will be responsible for making the necessary adaptations and changes in your life. You are the only one who can cooperate with cancer therapy and make any changes in behavior that might optimize your chances of survival.

If you're going to take responsibility for your part of coping with your cancer therapy and your recovery, you'll want to assert that you have a vital role to play in treatment decisions. Your active participation in your healthcare can make a big difference in your adjustment to your illness and possibly in its outcome.

Medical Training and Emotions

Dr. Rachel Naomi Remen writes in her book *The Human Patient*, "Expressing caring directly, rather than through a willingness to work a thirty-six hour day or a meticulous attention to the current literature, transgresses a strong professional code."

Before the recent technological advances in medicine and the routine use of X-rays, CT, and nuclear scans, doctors had to humbly acknowledge the limits of their craft and give credence to the patient's own ability to recover and heal. While there have been improvements, too many doctors fail to acknowledge, appreciate, and consider the emotions, beliefs, and subconscious strengths of their patients.

It isn't necessary to blame physicians for this failure, nor does it make sense to add another course to the already overburdened medical school curriculum. The point is that to be more scientific, doctors need to acknowledge that patients do have feelings, emotional reactions, and beliefs that can evoke stress responses and, therefore, affect the body's ability to heal. Patients also can learn skills to calm their bodies and improve the effectiveness of medical treatments.

A medical student, in good academic standing and highly thought of by his peers, dropped out of school during his second year because of what he felt is an inherent hypocrisy in medical training. Medical students are constantly subjected to an unhealthy mix of criticism, stress, and frequent humiliation. This, along with the pressure and the limited focus, make it an unhealthy environment and one unlikely to produce physicians who can show concern for the health needs of others. He writes:

> I felt that medical school was not training healers. It was training technicians who deal with disease ... I worked up an eighty-eight-year-old woman who had a lot of problems—all her organs were running down. She knew she was dying and didn't really want to be in the hospital. Mostly what she wanted was a back rub, and a nice place to just be and die. But she was tested for every disease in the book. As part of this she was put on a water-restricted diet, plus she was put on diuretics. She was lying in bed moaning. "I want water ..." So I gave her water. It made me see that this massive body of facts about disease was getting in the way of basic health care. The doctors would come in and look at her tumor or listen to her lung, but they would not listen to what she was saying about what she wanted. Nobody was.

Medical schools traditionally have not taught their future doctors how to listen to patients' concerns and emotions. In fact, they've taught medical students to fear their own emotions as something that might bias their objectivity. This argument assumes that feelings are not objective facts.

To become more scientific our medical schools will need to teach that emotions and beliefs are real, and that they can have an enormous impact on the patient's physical reactions and, therefore, on the patient's health. If you are not getting the care you wish, insist that your doctor be more scientific.

How to Take Charge of Your Medical Treatment

If you observe the way doctors and nurses manage their medical treatment you can learn a lot about maintaining control over your own healthcare. When doctors get sick they refuse to put up with the standard humiliations and discourtesies that you and I passively endure. They are notorious for being the worst patients on the ward.

Doctors and nurses are aware that the patient role in the typical doctor-patient relationship is one of diminished power, and so they fight hard to maintain some level of equality. Of course, doctors know the language of this medical country that is foreign to most of us, but more than that, they have ways of avoiding passivity and depersonalization. Doctors and nurses ask many questions about why a test or procedure has been ordered, often refuse to take tests they have not been informed about, and complain loudly when their rest is interrupted for the convenience of the hospital staff. Nor will they allow themselves to be intimidated into a procedure by the threat that if they refuse, their chart will include the notation, "acted against doctor's orders." In other words, it actually may be good for you to act like a doctor-patient and risk being labeled a "bad patient."

Be Prepared to Ask Questions

In the course of your experience with cancer, as a patient or as a relative, you will have many questions to ask your doctor. Often, however, you may not know which questions to ask and may even feel that you should not trouble the doctor. Your doctor might assume, therefore, that the information he or she has provided meets your needs or that you are afraid of hearing the diagnosis.

You may have to tell the doctor when you want more information, and the doctor may need to ask, "How much do you want to know?" Patients and their physicians must stop assuming that they can read each other's minds or interpret silence! Ask:

1. Doctor, what's your diagnosis of my illness?

2. If it's cancer, what type of cancer?

Ask for the spelling of the tumor's name and ask for its stage or level. You'll need this information when you do an online search and when you consult with another doctor for a second opinion.

3. If it's cancer, has it spread?

The doctor will tell you if the tumor has metastasized to the lymph nodes or lungs or if it is confined to one site (*in situ*).

4. What is the treatment plan you're following?

You could also ask for the research articles that support this protocol if you or family members want to get further information from a medical library or the Internet.

5. What are the alternative treatments and treatment schedules?

Alternative or adjunctive treatments may be available for your type of cancer. You also may be able to delay a treatment, without increased risk, a few days or weeks to complete your vacation plans or to obtain the opinions of other specialists.

6. What are the risks in waiting or doing nothing?

Some cancers, such as some prostate cancers, are slow-growing and a "wait-and-see" approach with periodic follow-up appointments could be an option.

7. What are the side effects, the risks, and the benefits of this treatment?

You might also tell your doctor, "If this is my best chance for survival I don't want to hear about the side effects. I just want my body to work with this medicine."

8. Why stage surgery first? Why not chemotherapy or radiation first to shrink the tumor or metastases?

The *staging* of treatments—such as using radiation before surgery to shrink the tumor—may be flexible for some cancers.

9. What will these tests determine? And what are the risks of doing these tests?

10. What is the purpose of this medication? What are the side effects, warnings, and interactions with other medications?

Let your doctor know of *all* the medications, supplements, and herbs you are taking. Often, they do not interact well with powerful medications.

11. Doctor, who do you recommend for a second opinion?

12. What can I do to help the treatment work for me and improve my chances?

Be prepared to ask these questions and whatever others will help you actively make it *your* treatment, something you know about, have a say in, and, therefore, can more easily cooperate with. You may want to invite a trusted friend or relative along when you see your doctor to ensure that you understand all the issues, and to assist you in asserting your rights and wishes.

If you get nervous asking your doctor questions, prepare your questions in advance in writing, checking them off as the doctor answers them. I encourage you to record or write down the doctor's responses and to ask for the correct spelling of medical terms and medications. Your doctor may be receptive to the use of a recorder, as Dr. Ernest Rosenbaum recommends in *Everyone's Guide to Cancer Supportive Care*. He suggests that recording your consultation with your doctor "enhances both the patient's and the family's understanding of the illness and therapy," and it "makes the physicians more conscious of the need for clarity" in their explanations.

Take Me Seriously—Respect My Feelings

The most common complaint I hear from patients about their doctors is, "They don't take me seriously; and they're annoyed if I get upset or scared." The most frequent positive statement made by patients about their doctors is, "He (or she) is patient and takes time to listen to my concerns."

Patients often feel that their worries might interfere with the doctor's work and are imposing on his or her busy schedule. It's only natural to want to keep the people treating you happy, especially when you feel so dependent on their attention and care. And trying to find another doctor is not always an option when time is of the essence and finances are limited.

Hospitals are run for the convenience of the medical staff, and, oddly enough, the patient's opinion is often not considered. You will want to break from this tradition. You have a right to ask your questions, even if they treat you as if you're emotional, elderly, or too young, irrational, or unaware of medical terminology. It's your body, and you're going to need to stand up and speak up for it!

Don't accept, "don't worry," as an answer. You may need to assert, "but doctor, I *am* worried, and I want to know what's wrong and what can be done." Let your doctors know that while you respect their opinions, you need to make your decisions based on your values, your feelings, and the facts currently available. You can let them know that you intend to participate in the decision-making, using their knowledge and skills to assist you, not to control you.

Medication

These days most hospitals will inform you of potential side effects of any medication you are given. But you may also want to know what results to expect, what instructions to follow, and any side effects that you should watch for. You have valuable input at this point because you know about your allergies, other medications you are taking, and your dietary and health habits.

Some medications and treatments are not recommended for certain conditions (such as pregnancy, liver disease, diabetes, and glaucoma), and many should not be combined with alcohol or caffeine. You need to inform your cancer specialist if any of these conditions apply. A physician unfamiliar with your medical history may neglect such important facts, especially when focused on the life-and-death aspects of your cancer treatment.

If you are hospitalized, you may also need the help of friends and family to make certain that each shift of nursing and hospital staff has read your chart. Without raising unnecessary fears, we all know of mistakes that have taken place in hospitals. The nurse on the night shift told one of my clients that it was time for her insulin injection for her diabetes. The patient had to insist several times that it was her roommate who was diabetic, not she. Be ready to refuse any medication that you're unfamiliar with.

Be sure to provide the staff with a list of the medications you are taking and any allergic reactions. Make multiple copies and make sure this list is in your chart.

As with the patient described above, if you are sharing a room with another patient, check to make sure you aren't being given a medication that belongs to that patient, and be especially vigilant about the night shift.

Use signs, lists, and whatever it takes to let them know that you will not take any medication that is not approved by your doctor and in your chart. One patient who was tired of being told to take the incorrect medication, wrote instructions on his stomach.

Make sure the hospital staff is familiar with your list of medications and allergic reactions before you agree to take any medication.

Protecting Yourself from Pessimism

When you've been shocked by the diagnosis of cancer, or are coming out of the anesthetic, you are particularly sensitive to negative or positive suggestions. All the conditions necessary for a hypnotic trance are present: You need and expect help, you see the doctor as an authority, you don't understand the medical procedures, and you are placed in a passive role from the time you enter the office and begin to follow orders.

Even if you don't think of yourself as vulnerable to suggestion, it probably makes sense to prepare yourself to take in only the healthy suggestions and to push away the negative.

Be aware of your own tendency to worry or panic and of your susceptibility to the attitudes, words, and actions of your doctors, nurses, and family. They can influence your own expectations of a good outcome or create stressful worry about a negative outcome.

Your relationship with your doctors and nurses throughout your therapy should be one that is supportive of your health and your emotional resilience. If you find their visits to be more upsetting than comforting, let them know that you want them to be sensitive to the effect their negative statements and attitudes have on you.

Here are some examples of negative statements that were said to my clients or me, "You will have a lot of pain. But don't worry we have medication we can give you." "It will take six months for you to recover." "Chemotherapy is highly toxic, and you will lose your hair and become nauseated."

Such statements predispose you to feeling pessimistic and depressed. More importantly, they take away the opportunity to lower your stress hormones and improve your healing process with statements such as:

> You will be receiving some very powerful medicine
> that is capable of killing rapidly producing cells. You
> may temporarily lose some hair because this medi-
> cine kills rapidly dividing cancer cells and, as a side
> effect, rapidly dividing hair cells. Fortunately, normal,
> healthy cells can recover from the treatment and re-
> produce themselves, but the weak, poorly formed
> cancer cells cannot. Your healthy hair will grow back.

This version gives you the opportunity to think of the chemotherapy as a powerful ally working to kill rapidly producing cells.
And the side effect of temporary loss of hair becomes evidence
that the medication is working. Moreover, the side effects are presented as possible, rather than definite, in order to avoid a self-
fulfilling prophesy.

Protecting yourself from pessimism involves several factors: an
awareness of your vulnerability to suggestion; recognition of the
bias of the speaker's perspective; and the ability to challenge nega-
tivism with your own positive concept of your body's ability to work
with and recover from medical treatments.

The Misuse of Statistics

Some doctors and nurses think that pessimism is more accurate,
more scientific, and more truthful than optimism. They are afraid
of giving their patients false hope. And, in the name of this fear,
they too often attempt to eradicate all reasonable hope with the
use of statistics. So be prepared for the inaccurate use of statistics and for your own misinterpretation of them. It's impossible to
place a statistic on the chances of survival for a single individual.
Statistics apply to the probabilities of group outcomes and only are
appropriate when describing a sample group. Even a guess at one
individual's chances must consider how that person compares to
the norm, and what unique physical and psychological resources
he or she possesses.

My doctor told me that I had a 10-percent chance to live one year if my cancer did not respond to chemotherapy. Fortunately, I knew something about statistics and was familiar with the research my oncologist was using to make his prediction. I knew that I was healthier, receiving better medical treatment, and living in a world two decades more advanced than most of the men in the sample from which he was quoting. Had I not had this advantage, I might have incorporated his misuse of statistics as the truth, and allowed it to dampen my hopes, efforts, and energy.

In all fairness to my doctor, I had asked him what my chances were. But the fact is, regardless of the probabilities for the overall group, my task (and yours) remains the same: to keep fighting for life until the moment when acceptance of death enhances the end of life. Whether you're given a 10-percent or a 90-percent chance to live, your job is the same; and if you are in the percentage that survives, you survive 100 percent!

For the most part, when a doctor answers a question about the chances of survival with a statistical probability, he or she is misunderstanding the patient and answering the wrong question. The doctor falls into the trap of trying to report on the latest research findings that included fifty or a thousand patients, with a variety of ages, stages of disease, and of unknown overall physical and mental health. In an attempt to answer what he or she thinks the patient is asking, the doctor, all too frequently, will make a grossly inaccurate use of statistics by offering to predict the chances of a specific individual.

A more humane and accurate answer to a patient's question about chances for survival would be the following:

> Each patient is different. Though I can calculate the stage of your disease, I cannot calculate the strength of your immune system or the power of your mind and body to rally when the going gets rough. I've seen patients pull through and outlive the odds. People with your type of cancer have had long-term remissions, some have lived with it for years, and some have died.

Your job is to maximize your chances and to do whatever you can for the healthy portion of your body. My job is to help you with the latest that modern medicine can offer. Let's work together and see what we can do to make you as healthy as possible.

Resources for Treating the Whole Patient

Your doctor is not the only medical resource or caregiver available to you on your healthcare team. You yourself are an important member of that team and are an essential resource. In order to maximize your chances of cooperating with your treatment and controlling or curing your cancer, you'll want to ask what you can do. Changes in your habits, smoking and drinking especially, and, perhaps, the reduction of fats and dietary improvement overall, could improve the quality of your life and your chances of remission and survival.

In order to have a complete treatment program to assist in your cancer therapy and to optimize the effects of your treatments, you might ask your doctor for a referral to a nutritionist or a medical social worker or psychologist. Remember, you're not just fighting cancer, you're supporting the 99 percent of your body that is healthy and the emotional-psychological parts of you that sustain your spirit on a difficult journey.

Nutrition and Cancer Therapy

Proper nutrition is another aspect of healthcare that is often undervalued in standard medical practice. Recent research indicates that nutritional support is beneficial to cancer patients, improves their response to chemotherapy and radiation therapy, and reduces side effects. You may find, however, that you have to initiate any discussion about nutrition and that your doctor may discount its importance. You, therefore, may want to see a nutritionist, or learn about a diet that is compatible with your treatment and your overall health needs. The maintenance of proper nutrition is one area where you and your family can have important and active roles in the overall fight against cancer.

You may find that radiation, chemotherapy, or psychological reactions leave you with loss of appetite. It can be extremely difficult to eat when the treatment, or food itself, makes you nauseated. But you can still learn to eat even when you don't feel like eating. You can learn to eat in order to:

1. Recover more rapidly from surgery

2. Lessen the side effects and improve your tolerance of radiation and chemotherapy

3. Improve the ability of your immune system to resist infection

4. Take an active role in your recovery from cancer

Psychosocial Support

A survey of doctors found only 20 percent believed that their patients wanted to talk about their personal or family problems. Yet 80 percent of the patients reported that they wished to discuss these issues.

Most cancer patients experience at least six periods during which psychosocial support could be of immense help. You may benefit from psychosocial support during each of these periods.

1. At the time of diagnosis—to help you understand and accept the diagnosis of cancer, how it can be treated, what treatment alternatives to consider, and to assist in communications within the family and with your doctors and nurses

2. In the preoperative period—to help you fully commit to surgery with less fear, anxiety, and stress

3. Following surgery—to assist in recovery and adjustment to any physical changes that may result from surgery, and to prepare you for any subsequent cancer therapy

4. During post-operative cancer therapy—to lessen your anxiety about tests and side effects, to lend support if there are any setbacks, and to aid in maintaining a sense of participation in your treatment so that any decisions to stop therapy can be made with medical advice, without jeopardizing the progress that has been made in suppressing or overcoming your cancer

5. At the completion of cancer therapy—to assist with rehabilitation, the transition from dependence on medication and the doctor to reliance on your own body, and with the establishment of a new self-image as a potentially healthy, active person

6. During the five-year follow-up period—to help you cope with a possible recurrence of cancer or fears about recurrence, with any long-term side effects of cancer therapy, and with your return to a life in which worry about cancer takes a backseat to your daily routines

During each of these periods, psychosocial support in the form of patient support groups, individual and family counseling, stress management, sexual counseling, and advice about jobs and finances, can facilitate adjustment and free your physical resources for the main task of recuperation and a return to health.

The Team Approach

One of the best ways of ensuring that your needs as a complete person are met during your cancer therapy is to enlist the help of a team of supportive services.

The presence of a team of experts acknowledges that you are a person with mental, emotional, social, and spiritual, as well as physical needs, and that no one individual can take responsibility for all of your needs. A cancer therapy team often includes the patient, the oncologist (usually a chemotherapist, radiation therapist, or surgeon), the primary or family physician, the nurse, the nutritionist, the medical social worker or psychologist, the physical or occupational therapist, and the chaplain or religious counselor.

A growing number of hospitals offer the team approach to cancer treatment and will offer you the opportunity to actively participate in your own recovery. Such programs clearly communicate that you are more than your disease, that you have a life beyond the hospital, and that they will not treat you like a helpless victim.

The team approach is not available in all hospitals, so unless you're willing to search for a doctor and a hospital that offer a holistic treatment of cancer patients—and it may be well worth your search—you can request the services of the supportive units available within your hospital or community. These services are usually available through the visiting nurse program, the hospital's psychiatry department, the medical social worker unit, or the hospital's religious counselors or chaplains.

Without supportive therapy, you may doubt the validity of your feelings and your need for something more than what the doctor offers. Some patients even feel embarrassed about having emotions that the doctor doesn't address. Your request for any of these services, however, may need to be cleared by the physician in charge, and this may result in a confrontation with your doctor. The benefits gained from having the validity of your emotional needs confirmed, however, is well worth the risk of rocking the boat.

The Nurse

Patients usually have a closer relationship with their nurses than they do with their doctors because nurses spend more time with the patient, touch the patient, and take time to listen to their questions and fears. The nurse is the one who helps with the daily challenges of recovery and preparation for treatment, administers drugs, changes dressings, and helps with personal needs such as use of the toilet, backrubs, change of bedding, and meals. Often nurses hear and see things that the doctor may miss. An oncology nurse told me of an incident which exemplifies the differences in perspective between doctors and nurses concerning their patients.

The doctor told the nurse that a particular patient was "in denial" because he didn't react to the doctor's presentation of a diagnosis of cancer. The nurse had a very different view. She had just spent a considerable amount of time soothing the patient and educating him about the favorable prognosis for his type of cancer and of the treatments that were available.

She informed the doctor that when the patient left his office he came to her crying, "I'm going to die." The patient perceived her as someone with whom he could cry, and she in turn was sympathetic, knowing the impact that the diagnosis of cancer can have on a patient.

This same nurse, Barbara (as I shall call her), often finds herself acting as an advocate for her patients. She does this by remaining in the room when the doctor arrives to make sure that the doctor answers the questions that the patient has asked her privately. When the patient forgets or is intimidated by the doctor, Barbara does a little coaching by saying, "Mrs. Jones wasn't there something else you wanted to ask the doctor?" or "Doctor, I believe Mrs. Jones has another question for you."

As with many nurses, Barbara frequently steers her patients away from insensitive doctors. "For example," she said, "I've seen the way some doctors do mastectomies, and I know the ones who take into consideration the cosmetic aspects and those who are unnecessarily aggressive during surgery." When she discovers that a patient has the latter type of doctor, she discreetly asks, "Of course, you're going to get a second opinion, aren't you?"

Your nurse can be the primary source of care giving for you and your family, turning the coldness of a large hospital into a warmer, more caring place. And it is the nurse who will often recommend that you seek a second opinion or referral to physical therapy, psychiatry, medical social work, home-visit nursing, or hospice. In this way the nurse provides you an opportunity to receive the full care you need to cope with the emotional impact of cancer.

Recommendations

1. Remember that, like all humans, your doctor, nurse, and medical staff can make mistakes. You, therefore, can take some responsibility for ensuring that you are getting the correct medication, that they are treating you for the correct disease, and that your doctors know of any information about your health and work habits that may affect your treatment.

2. Ensure that your needs for emotional support and for information on self-care are made known and, if necessary, that you are given referrals to people who can provide these important aspects of health care.

3. Be aware that doctors—and any specialists, for that matter—have a tendency to see their specialty (surgery, for example) as the primary treatment while downplaying the importance of other medical specialties and other health services. You, therefore, could benefit from contact with a primary care or family physician who can look after your overall health and coordinate the recommendations of the specialists, considering them in light of your medical and family history.

4. Assure your doctor that you can take responsibility for your body and your life. While some doctors might say that they are responsible for your life, you are the one who must follow through on medications and treatments, and it is you who will live with the side effects and benefits.

5. Speak up for the ability of your body to heal and maintain a balance between the helpful advances of modern science and the ancient wisdom of your body and mind. Don't let a limited, mechanistic view of medical science overrule or ignore the wisdom of your mind and the vitality of your body.

6. Assume that your doctors have good intentions and want to help. But, like all of us with good intentions, they sometimes

are too quick to impose their help before ascertaining what you need. Find a doctor who is open to hearing your needs and your perspective and who takes the time to listen.

7. Maintain the positive expectation that you will receive good care from your medical providers, and assume that it is your right as a patient.

8. Let your healthcare givers know when they deviate from good, humane medical care. Let them know if an attitude, a procedure, or a treatment is inhibiting your ability to calm your body and enhance its healing potential. Persist until your request reaches someone who is concerned about the total care of patients. Demand that the medical profession live up to its own high standards of good medicine and good patient care.

Chapter 8

Communication Skills:
Staying Connected

You may have learned that the words *cancer* and *cancer patient* carry with them a stigma, causing discomfort among many people. It's difficult enough for you to face the fear and helplessness of cancer without having to protect others from your feelings.

Communications within the Family

A serious illness will accentuate any communication problems that already exist in your family and can add stress to all your relationships. Relatives and friends may feel that talking about your illness is a threat to peace within the family, making the expression of your true feelings difficult. In addition to your own hesitation to talk about cancer, illness, and possibly death, your family and friends no doubt have their own reservations about discussing these issues that can block open communications.

The more extensive your cancer, the greater can be the barriers to communication. Doctors and nurses also can make it difficult for you to express concerns or ask questions, at times directing the conversation into "safe channels." Your need to express your feelings, however, is legitimate regardless of the reactions of your family or the medical staff. In fact, research has shown that those who express the uncomfortable feelings of depression and anger often cope better than those who try to suppress these feelings and attempt to be cheerful for the benefit of others.

If your family, friends, or doctors feel uncomfortable by your open communication of sadness, anger, or grieving, you could benefit from speaking to a professional therapist, medical social worker, or hospital chaplain. And if you, in spite of the comforting support of family, friends, or doctor find it difficult to talk about your feelings and concerns, you definitely could benefit from talking to a professional.

Regardless of your ability to communicate and express your feelings, the crisis of cancer will require sharpened skills and persistent effort in order to maintain the good relationships and support so important in coping with this illness.

Why Communicate Your Feelings?

Not only is the topic of cancer a difficult one to talk about, but, in this rugged individualist society of ours, you may have been trained to silently endure your fears and anger and to hide your hopes. Our skepticism about the usefulness of expressing emotions is reflected in such common statements as, "Just talking's not going to help me cope," and, "I don't want to burden others with my problems."

I know that, at times, I have kept things to myself. For example, when I received orders for Vietnam, I didn't tell anyone. I knew from Special Forces troops about the booby traps and mines that had killed or crippled their buddies. I was terrified, but I kept my fears inside, telling myself that I was protecting my family and friends from upset. But even then, I knew that I was really protecting myself. Part of me knew that if I started talking about it, I would see their fears and would lose control myself. I was afraid I would fall apart and cry, and maybe even let them know of what I feared could happen to me.

So I went on that plane in the middle of the night without any of my loved ones knowing where I was going or how I felt. I fooled myself into believing that I was being a hero by protecting them from feelings that I was too afraid to face myself.

Nine years later, when I got cancer, I knew I couldn't bear a repetition of that sad scene of false heroism. I knew I had to tell my family and friends. I wasn't going to bear this war alone! I had a strong sense that holding in my feelings would be detrimental to my body. I wanted to release as much stress as I could in order to free my body and mind to fight cancer.

Recently I learned that putting a gut reaction into words begins a higher brain process of problem solving that makes overwhelming feelings more manageable while lowering stress and anxiety. Expressing your thoughts and feelings releases physical tension, gives you a new perspective on your experience, and breaks through the isolation of bearing your emotions alone.

Expressing a New Identity

Most of your life you may have thought of yourself as healthy and in control. Suddenly you have cancer, and all those thoughts prove to be false assumptions. The experience of cancer has an impact, not only on your body, but also on your self-image and on your view of how the world is supposed to be.

It's as if the universe has gone crazy, and along with it, the very cells of your body. You might ask, "If I'm no longer the healthy, active, in-control person I thought I was, then who am I? How do I make sense of my place in a world where the rules suddenly seem foreign, unclear, and unpredictable?"

It's precisely at this time that a clear expression of what you feel and think becomes so essential in reestablishing a new sense of identity. Out of the confusion brought on by the loss of your old self, and heightened by thoughts of what should have happened and what should not have happened, evolves a new self based on what is—what you are thinking, experiencing, and feeling, now.

When you start saying, "this is how I feel," "I want to do this," and "I am worried about that," you are affirming who you are. Having cancer makes it imperative that you express thoughts such as these:

- This is the way I feel

- This is what I am thinking

- This is what I really want

- I have no time for denying who I am and how I feel

- I want to grasp every moment as it presents itself, without fretting over how I should be, should feel, or should think

Choosing How to Communicate

Speaking, writing, drawing, singing, and labeling your thoughts and feelings during a crisis allows you to stand back and observe your reactions to an otherwise overwhelming experience. As a part of yourself observes, identifies, and categorizes your reactions, you gain control over them and realize that you are more than your thoughts and feelings. You are the one who can now decide which thoughts and feelings to act on, which to let go of, and which to examine further.

Perhaps this is one reason so many patients with cancer write and speak about their experience with the hope that it will be of use to others. The simple act of acknowledging thoughts and feelings and putting them out there where they can be looked at and heard, makes them less frightening and overwhelming. Written down or spoken, they become simply thoughts and feelings that you, from a calm perspective, can let go of or decide how to act on.

As you begin to observe your thoughts and choose which ones to express, you can begin to notice the degree to which your reactions are based on your beliefs and attitude and only partially on the actual events of your life. You can have all sorts of bizarre thoughts and never once act on them, but acknowledging them puts you in touch with the varied facets of your experience as a human being—love, fear, anger, tenderness, sexuality, and curiosity. Then you can decide which facets of your multifaceted personality to actualize in the world.

Speaking the Unspeakable

In groups I've led for cancer patients and their families, the issue that surfaces as the most pressing—after the shock of the diagnosis and the stress of coping with cancer therapy—is how to communicate with doctors and family. Whenever I ask group members about problems with their interpersonal communications, approximately 75 percent initially say, "there's no problem." But on reflection, the patient, a relative, or both, will acknowledge that often it's not so easy to talk about what's really on their minds.

The relatives of the patient often feel that the patient considers certain topics taboo. Patients, on the other hand, often feel that if they allow themselves to get upset, everyone else will become hysterical. The patients then feel they have to suppress their own feelings in order to take care of the rest of the family. Soon it becomes obvious that everyone has become overly cautious about bringing up certain topics.

What gradually emerged from these groups was a series of statements that are particularly effective in initiating discussions of uncomfortable thoughts or feelings. While many of these statements might be helpful to either the patient or the family, the first two are primarily from the patient's perspective and the rest are from the point of view of the family.

- I'm afraid that my cancer has made us strangers. I'm feeling increasingly isolated and alienated from you, as if we're going through our own private hells separately. Is there anything that I can do to help you through this time? We've become so tentative with each other, lately. Can't we find a way to really talk?

- I'm finding it very difficult to tell you of my feelings about this illness, this cancer. And I'm afraid that if I bring it up you'll get upset.

- You know, some things are really hard to think about,

much less talk about. And I just want you to know that if you ever want to talk to me about them, I'm more than willing to listen.

- I feel bad about avoiding talking to you about all the troubles you've been going through. I'm afraid that if we start talking I'd break down and cry, and you wouldn't like that.

- You seem really calm about all this, so I've tried not to get you upset with my feelings. But I'm really scared about losing you.

- Please don't tell me not to worry. I am worried, and with good reason. This is serious! And I get very upset when you make jokes about it, and tell me there's nothing to worry about. I don't want to lose you.

- Let's figure out what we're going to do if the test comes back positive. I'm hoping for the best, but I'd feel a lot better if I knew what you were thinking and what we'll do if it turns out to be bad news.

What the Family Can Say

In spite of all the good intentions and efforts on the part of the family, at times the patient seems to be resisting all efforts to talk seriously about the illness. Under such circumstances there's not much to do but to trust the patient's way of coping and to let him or her know that when it's time to talk, you'll be there. This kind of support can be vital to a patient who's waiting for a sign that somebody cares. You might say it like this:

I want to talk to you, but I get the feeling that there are some things you'd rather not talk about now. I want you to know that when you're ready to talk, I'm ready to listen. I won't turn away if you cry, and I hope you won't mind if I cry. I want you to have someone to share your thoughts and feelings with, if you want to. If I were in your place, the worst thing would be feeling isolated from my friends. I don't want you to feel that way. We've shared some good times; we can share this too.

If you can't imagine yourself actually saying these things out loud, you may want to write down your thoughts in a note. Writing down difficult feelings enables you to complete your message without the fear of interruption. It also allows you to make as many changes as you need in order to accurately express how you feel.

Three Barriers to Communication

The inability to talk about your problems and feelings is a most serious obstacle to having a good relationship. Every relationship has its problems, but if you can talk about them you have a better chance of living through them, together. It makes sense, especially during times of serious illness, to be aware of barriers to open communications. In my work with cancer-stricken families I have seen three major barriers to communication: a conspiracy of silence, premature mourning, and a need to be heroic.

A Conspiracy of Silence

With any serious illness and emotional topic, there is the danger of avoiding mentioning it for fear of saying the wrong thing and evoking strong feelings. This can lead to a conspiracy of silence in which the patient and the family avoid the topic in an attempt to protect each other, all the while creating feelings of alienation, misunderstanding, and barriers to direct and open communication.

Out of a sense of duty and a desire to protect a loved one, a vicious cycle of silence, misinterpretation, guesswork, and isolation gets started. Phrases like, "I don't want to say anything because I'm afraid she'll get upset," or "They haven't brought it up so I assume they just don't want to talk about it," are signs that a conspiracy of silence is taking place.

While you want to respect another's timing, this doesn't mean that you must sit silently with your own feelings and try to interpret clues as to when it's okay to speak. You can still invite a conversation with phrases such as, "I don't know what to say but I want you to know that I'd be glad to talk whenever you wish," or "Please let me know when you'd like to talk about what you've been through."

We cannot protect others from reality; they usually have some idea of what's going on and often are imagining the worst. Even though our intentions are good, the desire to protect someone from hurt usually comes with an attempt to protect ourselves from our own upset. It generally makes sense to say something about what is troubling you, even if you choose to keep the details vague. For example, "I've been avoiding talking to you because I've been afraid I'd break down and cry. If you don't mind me crying, I'd be glad to talk with you." Let them know that you can handle your own emotions and that you don't need protection from their feelings. If the two of you are going to cry, at least you can cry together.

Premature Mourning

Learning that a loved one has cancer often causes family members to start a painful premature mourning process and to be less available to support the patient's ongoing treatments. Anticipating that you'll have to repeat the mourning process in the future can lead to avoidance of the patient, thereby depriving the patient of real, human contact. Patients and their families and friends have different timetables for grieving and adapting to how cancer has affected them.

Even when we know that many forms of cancer are curable, there remains the fear that a cancer diagnosis is a death sentence. This fear can lead us to mourn the loss of a loved one even though he or she may recover from cancer, may live with it for years, or may want to enhance the quality of the last months of life with frequent visits and support from family and friends.

Of course, the patient can be the one who's doing the premature mourning, isolating himself from the family and depriving them of an opportunity to share feelings and to express their concern and desire to help.

Please remember that being diagnosed with cancer, having cancer, and dying of cancer are separate and different states, each requiring its own emotions and adjustments, each in its own time. Eventually, the premature mourner must cope with the present moment rather than the imagined future. The patient may want to tell the premature mourner what I told a friend:

> Stop avoiding me and treating me as if I'm already dead. I'm still here. I'm still alive! I need you to be with me, now. Help me to make the most of whatever time is left. There'll be plenty of time for grieving after I'm gone. But don't be so sure I'm going that fast. In fact, I may hang around so long that you may be saying, "How can I miss you if you won't go away?"

You most likely will find that, as you become more comfortable with these difficult feelings, you'll worry less and will enjoy more fully the valuable time that you still have with each other.

The Need to Be Heroic: A Refusal to Mourn

The need to be a heroic helper, strangely enough, can get in the way of hearing what the patient needs and wants from you. Communication breaks down when you focus on your own agenda rather than on listening to the needs of the other person.

When my mother first learned she had cancer, I wanted to make sure that she was getting the best treatment possible, that all the appropriate tests were administered, that all the precautions were taken, and that a second opinion was considered. Keeping myself in a frenzy, I contacted everyone I knew who might have information about her type of cancer and its treatment. I went to medical libraries and copied pages of diagnostic procedures, treatments, and the research indicating the chances for a cure. I was relentless in bugging the doctors to insure they were doing the right thing. I felt this tremendous compulsion to help, but it wasn't clear how this would be useful to my mother. I became concerned that much of my need seemed to come out of a desire to feel powerful in the face of so much helplessness.

Of course, I wanted to do whatever I could to help my mother, but I had to be careful that my own need to conquer cancer and protect her from pain, didn't rob her of her independence. The exaggerated sense of responsibility and protection that I felt came out of my own need to be helpful and, possibly, heroic. I reminded myself that it is her life and that she must be in control. I could offer advice, but she had to decide what to do. Her style of coping with illness was very different from my own and needed to be heard and respected.

Without blaming yourself, be aware that your initial reaction to the illness of a friend or family member may be frenetic activity to escape the helplessness that often accompanies it. Some portion of this activity may be useful in gathering information that reassures you that the doctor is informed of the latest and best procedures.

Accepting Yourself and the Patient as Human

When someone close to you is seriously ill, it is only natural to feel that life is suddenly out of your control. Not only are you helpless to prevent your loved one from being stricken with a serious illness, you also must acknowledge that you're equally vulnerable to the same thing happening to you. As if it's not enough that you're dealing with a threat of losing someone you love, you also have to face your own fears of vulnerability to illness, helplessness, and death.

Cancer, and the cancer patient can become, therefore, unwelcome reminders of your own humanness, vulnerability to disease, and mortality. If you don't face your own fears and limits, you may unwittingly perceive the patient as a threat to your delusion of being a superhuman who's invulnerable to illness. You may find that you want to avoid your sick friend, and may even become angry with them for not getting better under your care.

Your well-intended desire to be helpful can lead to a need to be heroic by rescuing the patient from cancer and the discomforts of medical therapies. It's difficult at this point to accept that you are not a god or an angel that can cure the world of cancer and serious illness.

Mourning the loss of childhood magical thinking and heroic roles is a major life task. But it is one that will teach you to accept yourself as human, with human limits, and human vulnerabilities and lead to inner peace. Refusing to let go of your childhood belief in magical powers can keep you stuck in frustration, anger, and guilt.

You don't have to stamp out cancer or pain in order to help your friend or family member. More than likely, the patient needs more mundane things from you—your time and friendship, help with shopping, and ten minutes of sharing human fears and feelings.

The importance of sensitive helping and communication is conveyed in the following story, told to me by the late Dr. Milton H. Erickson about how his two daughters, ages five and eight, cared for their older brother when he was sick.

> Whenever this unusually active and vibrant boy was sick, he secluded himself from the rest of the family and slept until the illness had passed, wanting nothing better than to be left alone. His eight-year-old sister admired her older brother very much, however, and wanted to take care of him. When he was sick, she was eager to offer him soup, books to read, things to talk about, and lots of questions about how he felt. The boy reluctantly accepted his sister's gifts and expression of caring, but tried to ignore her so he could go back to sleep. After a while, however, his fatigue and illness got the best of him, and he yelled at her to leave him alone, causing hurt feelings all around.

The five-year-old sister quietly observed how her older sister tried to help. But, she didn't know how to make soup, and her books were of no interest to her older brother. She wasn't sure what she could do for him that would make him feel better. This didn't stop her from finding her own way of expressing caring that was more in keeping with his needs.

She took her favorite stuffed bear and, without disturbing her brother, placed it where he could reach it from his bed if he needed it. On awakening from his sleep, the boy saw his little sister's gift, and tears welled up in his eyes. She had understood.

Three Essential Communication Skills

Once you're aware of the barriers to effective communications and of ways of expressing complex emotions, you may want to apply three essential communication skills: framing, listening, and assertiveness.

These skills can be useful at any time in your life, but they are essential at times like these, when so much stress is being placed on your relationships.

Framing Difficult Feelings

When you "frame" difficult feelings, you include all the feelings, the initial anxiety as well as the fear of hurting someone. In the situations that follow, notice that several feelings are superimposed. For example, the patient may be angry but hesitant to express that anger for fear of hurting a close friend. In such situations it can help to frame your feelings in order to make it easier to express all the conflicting feelings. Here is an example of how one might frame this patient's feelings:

This is difficult for me to say because I really value your friendship, and I'm afraid you'll misunderstand

and get hurt. But the truth is, I'm really angry at you
for not coming to visit me in the hospital.

This patient has communicated several feelings: how difficult it is for him to bring up the topic; that he values the relationship; his fear of hurting the other person; and his feelings of anger.

It might be very difficult in this situation to say, "I'm really angry at you," and that would not communicate the feeling of caring for your friend and the relationship. These conflicting feelings along with the hurt make it almost impossible to simply say, "I'm angry." Sensing your difficulty, the person you're trying to communicate with might misinterpret your nonverbal signs of nervousness.

Fortunately, you don't have to build up the courage to express a difficult feeling. You can place your feelings of hurt and anger within the frame of the other emotions of caring and concern for the relationship.

In his book *Notes to Myself*, Hugh Prather examines the problem of expressing conflicting feelings. After thinking it through, he concludes that he has more than just his initial negative feeling.

> I thought that I was stuck with the feelings I had, that I couldn't change them, and shouldn't try even if I could. I saw many negative feelings inside me that I didn't want, and yet I felt that I must express them if I were going to be myself.

> Since then I have realized that my feelings do change and that I can have a hand in changing them. They change by my becoming aware of them. When I acknowledge my feelings they become more positive. And they change when I express them. For example, if I tell a man I don't like him, I usually like him better.

If we apply framing to Hugh Prather's dilemma, it might go something like this, "I have this negative feeling that I'm not very comfortable with. Yet I don't want to deny that it's part of me. Maybe if I tell you that I have this negative feeling toward you, it will change."

Framing your feelings is usually preferable to trying to hide them. You cannot not communicate. If you try to hide your feelings, friends will try to interpret (often misinterpreting) what you're feeling. When you're finding it difficult to communicate your thoughts and feelings, consider writing them out and putting them within the frame of your more positive feelings. You'll soon discover the relief that comes from being able to accurately communicate to your friends and family.

Active Listening

Our culture is so strongly oriented toward rapid problem solving that we have trouble simply listening to problems and emotions without attempting to offer a solution. When we give advice and offer solutions, however, we run the risk of insulting the listener by implying that their problem is simple and has an obvious solution that they have failed to see. By prematurely jumping to solutions, we tend to communicate impatience for their pain, and an unwillingness to share with them the unpleasant reality of their present condition.

When you're having difficulty communicating with a loved one, both of you may be trying to problem solve or win an argument rather than listen to each other.

When we try to help others, we tend to give advice, point out their mistakes and flaws in logic, and attempt to convince them that they can easily change their behavior if they would only try. This kind of help leads the listener to defend herself and to argue that the behavior isn't so bad, that we're just being too picky, and that we don't understand the special problems that lead her to resort to the behavior in the first place. We then are caught in an endless circle of good intentions followed by defensive behavior that often degenerate into accusations. And all of this started with an attempt to help.

If you remember that the primary goal of communication is understanding, much of this frustration can be avoided. The goal is not to give her advice. When she tells you, "Yes, but you don't understand," you'll know that you are giving advice before you have properly listened and demonstrated that you understand her problem. The frequency of her "yes, buts" will indicate that you should stop trying to help by giving advice and return to just listening.

We cannot always solve the problems of others or remove their pain, but we can listen, share, and understand. Ironically enough, out of this understanding comes a new solution—a sense of support that gives us the courage to continue through the times of suffering—without having to remove the problem.

More sensitive listening is a skill that can be learned. If you and a partner follow these steps, you will be able to discuss most topics to the point where you achieve mutual understanding. Participants in my groups have found that the more sensitive the topic and the more heated the discussion, the more they needed some guidelines for achieving satisfactory communication. They have learned that the process of accurate and active listening flows more naturally after using the following guidelines once or twice.

1. Schedule a time when the two of you can talk without interruption.

2. Face each other so that you are able to observe facial expressions and body language. Leave enough room between you to be comfortable; experiment with three to four feet of space. Avoid placing any furniture between you.

3. Decide who will speak first. While one speaks, the other actively listens and observes. The listener concentrates on the speaker's words, tone of voice, and body language, in order to be able to paraphrase the total message. The speaker stops after five to ten sentences or after one complete idea—just enough time for the listener to grasp the meaning, and short enough to permit paraphrasing.

4. The listener paraphrases the words and observable expressions of the speaker, without interpretation or correction. If the speaker is going too fast, the listener can interrupt and say: "Wait a minute. Let me see if I understand what you've said so far."

5. After the listener has paraphrased the words, the speaker points out where the listener was accurate, corrects any miscommunication, and shares any insights gained from hearing how his or her verbal and nonverbal message was perceived.

6. The process continues until the first speaker is finished and satisfied that he or she is understood. Then the speaker and listener change roles (changing seats is a good idea, too) and repeat the process until the second speaker has completed his or her message.

Paraphrasing requires careful attention to the speaker's words, tone, and physical messages, as well as to the selection of words that capture the feeling and meaning of the communication. The objective is to feed back to the speaker the essence of what he or she communicated verbally and nonverbally. Paraphrasing serves the following purposes:

- It focuses the listener's attention on the speaker rather than on judging, debating, or seeking solutions.

- It conveys to the speaker respect and a sincere effort to try to understand.

- It provides the listener with a check on the accuracy of his or her perceptions.

- It assists the speaker in clarifying the meaning, as well as exploring new meanings, of the feelings communicated. An example of paraphrasing for this purpose would be, "Your words stated that you feel hurt, but your tone of voice and clenched fist make me wonder if you're also angry."

After you've followed the guidelines completely at least once, you can use them flexibly, but stick to the essence of listening to each other rather than debating. Families who have used listening skills have been amazed at how helpful they can be in unraveling intricate blocks to communication and mutual understanding.

Assertiveness

Assertiveness gives you the ability to communicate difficult feelings without threatening or disparaging others, without violating your own values of courtesy and self-control, and without surrendering your self-respect.

The difficulty in communicating with busy and respected physicians, as well as with pressured receptionists, nurses, and administrators, is compounded if the only tool you have for the expression of strong feelings is aggression. You are even less likely to get what you want if you always rely on being passive.

Both aggressiveness and passivity limit the effectiveness of your communication. They are both aspects of the same attitude toward life. They both come from a win-lose or competitive model of life in which someone must give up something in order that another can win or feel good. The passive person often believes that if he's patient and nice enough, he'll eventually get what he wants. This attitude results in frequent experiences of being stepped on, justifying occasional outbursts of aggressiveness, followed by guilt and a return to passivity. The aggressive person feels that in a win-lose model of the world, he's going to win by do the stepping first. Occasionally he feels guilty and finds someone to step on him, thereby validating his view of life and justifying his return to aggressiveness.

This win-lose model of life comes from the belief that everyone is a potential threat to your self-worth. It can be exhausting to maintain this approach to life—you must always be on the lookout, always ready for a fight. Assertiveness, on the other hand, advocates a no-lose model of life in which two or more points of view can coexist without destroying or invalidating each other.

The basic principle of assertiveness is that it is not necessary to be better than the other person in order to maintain your self-respect or to firmly hold your ground. You are here, and you have a right to be here—as much right as the trees and the stars. You are made to survive—with each cell in your body and brain fighting for your survival—and to thrive in this life. You don't need to justify your existence to anyone.

Furthermore, your self-worth and self-respect can't be earned with intelligence, power, wealth, strength, or beauty. No one and nothing can give you a sense of self-worth. You are the only one who can allow yourself to discover an innate worth that is part of your birthright. From the assertiveness point of view, it is possible to hold your ground when someone is pressuring you or using aggressive tactics. The following are some examples of assertive statements that can be used in such situations:

- I cannot give you an answer right now; I will need time to make up my mind.

- You have made some excellent points, and you are very convincing, but I don't want to argue, and I have my own reasons for not wanting to do it.

- You are a better debater than I am, and you have obviously thought a lot about this issue, but I have my own plans.

When an aggressive person is arguing, he usually implies that because of your ignorance, guilt, low social status, or inability to debate, you should give them what they want, even if it's at your expense. You can counter this kind of argument by making it clear that your self-worth is not an issue for their judgment, and that your power is not based on any debatable standard. Your self-worth and your rights are never the issue as long as you refuse to let them be judged. You can deflate their argument further by even admitting to being insufficiently prepared to debate them, and still hold that, with all your imperfections, you have a right to your own opinion.

It is my belief that assertiveness comes from an attitude that self-worth is a birthright for every human being, regardless of ability or status, and from recognition that all points of view are subjective and incomplete maps of reality. Given that no one can know the objective truth, it makes sense to consider all points of view and to add these observations of reality so as to improve your own subjective map.

In the parable of the blind men who come upon an elephant, each argues that he knows what an elephant truly is. One has the tail and argues that an elephant is like a rope; another has a leg and argues that an elephant is like a tree; and so on. Each has an incomplete view of what constitutes an elephant. If they would stop arguing that one view must be right and all others wrong, they would be able to assemble a more accurate description of an elephant. This would require them to listen to each other, respecting the others' points of view while maintaining the validity of each point of view. Rather than saying, "I'm right and you're wrong," a more assertive response would be, "I understand that your experience tells you that an elephant is like a rope, while my experience tells me that an elephant is like a tree. Before we assume that we both can't be correct, let's consider the possibility that we are both partially correct."

Rather than pointing an accusing finger and saying such things as, "You are wrong," or "You make me angry," an assertive response uses "I-statements." ("I think," "I prefer," and "I feel" are the most common forms of I-statements." They help to present your statement as being simply your point of view, making them less threatening to the other person's view of reality, because they do not accuse or argue. Saying "I feel hurt when you don't come to see me," will get you a very different response than, "You are insensitive and selfish."

Saying "You're insensitive and selfish," puts the other person on the defensive, starts a debate, and doesn't deal with the issue. A more assertive statement might be, "I feel lonely when you don't visit," or "I'd prefer it if you'd visit me on the weekend," or "I feel neglected, and I'm starting to feel resentful."

The attitude and techniques of assertion training can also be of use to cancer patients and their families whenever it is necessary to say no. In such situations it is best to acknowledge the other person's feelings while at the same time asserting your own. Assertive statements that empathize with another's feelings usually begin as follows: "I can understand that you're feeling … " or, "I recognize that you want … " or, "I can hear that you … " Here are a couple of examples.

- I understand that you want very badly to talk with me right now, and I wish I were feeling up to it. But this isn't a very good time for me. I'd prefer to talk when I'm feeling stronger and can give you my full attention.

- I realize that you're very busy, and you have other patients to attend to. So, I won't take much of your valuable time, but I'd like to talk soon about something that's upsetting me.

When you assert your wishes you can always maintain your self-respect, whether or not you get what you want. In one sense, you never lose. At the very least, you've made your opinion known. These techniques are self-reinforcing because when you use them, you communicate what you want in a nonthreatening way, increasing your chances of achieving your goal. You focus on the real issues, lessening time wasted in needless and hurtful arguments.

Assertiveness fits well with the other essential communication skills of framing and active listening. All three support each other in helping you maintain more effective and open relationships with your doctors and family. Framing, active listening, and asserting will also assist you in the maintenance of your self-worth while avoiding conflict and defensiveness with others.

As with the other coping skills in this book, these skills have an additional purpose of freeing more of your energy for the maintenance of your physical health during this very stressful time. As you practice these skills, you will find that they help you become more effective in the world and in your relationships, and that they are powerful allies in a battle with cancer or any serious illness.

Different Timetables—Different Tasks

One of the reasons why communication becomes complex for you and your family is that you each have a different timetable for adapting to the cancer crisis. It's quite common for one person—the patient, for example—to quickly think through the issues of surgery, follow-up treatment, and even the possibility of dying of cancer. Others in the family may still be at the stage of disbelieving the diagnosis, seeking a second opinion, and worrying about the possible death of the patient.

Patients and family members also have different tasks of adjustment. The patient will face the shock of the diagnosis and then must quickly make decisions about life-saving treatment procedures. The family most likely will experience feelings of helplessness about being unable to save a loved one from the fear of cancer, the pain of medical treatment, and possibly death.

These differences in tasks and timing add to the difficulty of clear communications. The patient, for example, may have decided that he or she is satisfied with a particular doctor while the family may want to continue the search for "the best possible care." This can lead to unwanted pressure on the patient and the accusation that he or she is not fully committed to fighting cancer. Mutual understanding of these different tasks, needs, and timetables within a family can facilitate the open expression of feelings which is so helpful in reducing the stress and pain of this experience.

Changes in Family Roles

The presence of cancer puts unique pressure on the stability of the roles family members play. The role the cancer patient played in the family is often left vacant, at least temporarily, as the patient assumes a new role, perhaps a more dependent, or withdrawn, or demanding and forceful role. Others in the family will feel pressure as they shift their roles to fill the gap.

Usually this is not a problem for those families that can be flexible about their role assignments and choices. In fact, many families rally in extraordinary ways to this challenge—the quiet member becoming outspoken, the rebel pitching in and cooperating. A real crisis can occur, however, when family members are unable to adjust to the demands of their new roles, or find it difficult to accept the new role played by the patient. Most families are unprepared for the emotional stress of having a loved one incapacitated, even temporarily. Maintaining the rights of the family, an area often neglected in cancer care, can help minimize conflict and the breakdown of communication within the family.

The Rights of Family Members

Friends and relatives of a patient with cancer may want to demonstrate their concern and caring by sacrificing much of their time and energy to help the patient in whatever way they can. But, eventually, they may be overwhelmed by the enormity of the task. They may also find that secretly they begin to resent the feelings of helplessness that can come from trying to help a loved one overcome cancer and the discomforts caused by cancer treatment.

Family and friends may even begin to wish for an immediate and clear solution—a total cure, or even death—to end the patient's suffering. Many family members have been distressed to find themselves saying, "When is he going to die? Why does the suffering and the waiting have to go on for so long?"

Though this is to be expected when the waiting becomes intolerable, there are ways to avoid ever reaching such a state of desperation. One way is to maintain your own life and your own goals as much as possible, realizing that no amount of sacrifice on your part is going to reverse cancer. Your sacrifice, however, might lead to unfortunate feelings of resentment. Do what you willingly wish to do without endangering your own health.

Whenever possible, a family can avail itself of professional help from nurses, the American Cancer Society, psychologists, and medical social workers to help lessen the burden of caring for the patient. A support group for cancer patients and their families, Make Today Count, has recognized the need to acknowledge the rights of family members and the need for the maintenance of stable routines within the family. Patients and relatives from the San Diego chapter participated in drawing up the following "Bill of Rights for the Friends and Relatives of Cancer Patients."

> *The relative of a cancer patient has the right and obligation to take care of his own needs. Even though he may be accused of being selfish, he must do what he has to do to keep his own peace of mind, so that he can better minister to the needs of the patient.*

> *Each person will have different needs .... These needs must be satisfied. The patient will benefit, too, by having a more cheerful person to care for him. The relative may need help from outsiders in caring for the patient. Although the patient may object to this, the relative has the right to assess his own limitations of strength and endurance and to obtain assistance when required .... If the patient attempts to use his illness as a weapon, the relative has the right to reject that and to do only what can reasonably be expected of him.*

> *If the cancer patient's relative responds only to the genuine needs of the moment—both his own needs and those of the patient—the stress associated with the illness can be minimized.*

As family members and the patient practice the skills of clear communications, the needs of each can be heard and respected, allowing for greater closeness.

Chapter 9

Fully Alive after Cancer—
The Transformative Power of
Facing a Life-Threatening Crisis

The survivors were not supermen; they were ordinary individuals ... living proof of the indomitable will of human beings to survive and of their tremendous capacity for hope .... If [Holocaust] survivors could somehow deal with their problems, they may serve as a model for all individuals who have gone through a crisis, be it a life-crippling disease, a debilitating accident, financial ruin, social ostracism, or the loss of loved ones.

—William Helmreich, *Against All Odds*

The Essential Lesson

What's astounding about crisis survivors isn't that they possessed special traits before their tragedy; it's that afterwards—burdened by innumerable losses, changes, and adjustments—they find meaning in their lives. Even if you are a survivor of only the diagnosis and early stages of cancer, you also can discover that within yourself there's resilience to adversity and a passion to live fully the remainder of your life.

As you, hopefully, join the ranks of the more than 65 percent who survive cancer, you too can learn to expand your life to include greater joy and a stronger, more compassionate sense of self. When you meet other cancer survivors, you will discover that despite past failures, shortcomings, or handicaps, extreme challenges can bring to light resources you never knew you had.

Learning to be fully alive after cancer may require a number of steps or may happen all at once for you. Survivors generally speak of four parts to the process: transforming your perspective on life, focusing on the present, mourning and releasing the past, and shifting out of former roles.

Transformation—New Potential for Cancer Patients

While you're in the midst of coping with the cancer diagnosis, treatment decisions and adjustments to side effects, it's difficult to imagine any benefit coming from the experience of cancer. Yet those who have written and spoken of their survival experience often tell of the positive changes that have taken place in their outlook and character as a result of facing the challenges of cancer.

A crisis, whether it relates to your health, a natural disaster, or your finances, requires you to dig deeper into your resources, change your beliefs about what's important in life, and can awaken a new passion for life. Though unwelcomed, a crisis gives you an opportunity to replace ineffective methods of coping with healthier, more balanced ways of managing work, family, and life challenges.

Because a crisis forces you to function outside the box of your usual abilities, it can serve as a powerful catalyst for dramatic change. Cancer had that effect on Valerie, a thirty-year-old breast cancer survivor, quoted by Deborah Hobler Kahane in her book, *No Less a Woman*:

> … life is finite and can't be predicted. It could be cancer or it could be the truck coming around the bend, and so some effort has to be made to wake up and live a day, every day, as if it matters …. It just isn't the same anymore. Because of that, all kinds of things become possible.

The realization that life is finite causes a major shift in perspective, and awakens in you a drive to make this day and this life of yours matter. New possibilities are now open to you because, during a disaster, your instinctive drives take over and you cope at your optimal levels to survive. In such moments, you may discover that you transcend your familiar and customary patterns of fear and self-doubt and unleash an inner strength you never knew you had.

Of course, not everyone who survives cancer is able to use it as a turning point in his or her life. A crisis such as cancer may also revive old fears and cause frustration about the need for medical treatment, changes in your plans, and limits on your life and activities.

Yet, Dr. Charles Garfield, author of *Peak Performance*, noticed that most cancer patients tend to become peak performers in order to cope with the impact of cancer. Garfield says that, like the peak performing athletes he studied, those diagnosed with cancer learn to focus on what they can do in the present moment, regardless of past failures or anticipated hardships. They learn the power of bringing their minds into this moment—the only moment there is to act effectively.

The Power of Living in the Present

A life-threatening illness may, at least temporarily, lessen many of your freedoms, activities and abilities, affecting what you *can't* do. All the more reason you will want to assert what you *can* do. By focusing on what you can do now, you release energy for productivity and recuperation that may be stuck in regrets about the past and anxiety about the future. Think of this release of energy like a Karate punch delivered by a black-belt martial artist who refuses to be overwhelmed by his attackers, whether imagined or real.

As you enhance your ability to savor and energize the present moment, you may find greater comfort and deep feelings of calm and peace. You might notice that you can quickly reduce stress by practicing a simple mindfulness exercise of three-part breathing in which you imagine that each exhalation releases upset about the past and allows you to float down into the support that's available in the present. Think of the chair, the floor, or the bed as symbols of external support and your autonomic nervous system as internal support, available whenever you exhale and release muscle tension. You can also practice rapidly exhaling—like a Karate shout—thoughts about the future and create a safe place in the present that is a brief vacation from worry.

With repeated daily practice you'll train your brain to bring your attention out of the past and the imagined future and into the present where your body can release energy for action.

Centering Exercise

Centering is a one-minute, twelve-breath exercise that transitions your mind from fretting about the past and future to focusing in the present—where your body must be. Centering in the present clears your mind of regrets about the past and worries about anticipated problems in the so-called future.

As you withdraw your thoughts from these imagined times and problems, you release yourself from guilt about the past and worry about the future. You experience a stress-free vacation in the present. You automatically tap into this state whenever you give way to moments of joyful abandon in play, the easy flow of creativity, or effortless performance.

Use this exercise each time you start a project, transition to another task or place, or prepare for a medical procedure or treatment. Within just a few weeks of daily practice, your body will learn to let go of muscle tension with each exhalation; your mind will learn to focus on the one task of accepting the healing support of the chair or the bed. Your brain-wave frequencies will lower in just a few moments to the recuperative, restful, and reparative levels of rapid eye-movement (REM) sleep.

1. Begin by taking three slow breaths, in three parts: one, inhale; two, hold your breath and tense your muscles; three, exhale slowly and float down into the support of chair, the floor, or the bed.

With each exhalation let go of the last telephone call, email, or commute and feel the support of whatever is holding you now. With your next exhalation accept that support, allowing your muscles to release any unnecessary tension. Let go of all thoughts and images about work and worry from the past. Clear your mind and your body of all concerns about what should have or shouldn't have happened in the past. Let go of old burdens and trying to fix old problems and other people. Let each exhalation be a signal to let go of the imagined past and to float down into the sensations of this moment, and your mind will be with your body in the only time there is, the present.

Say to yourself as you exhale, "I release my mind and body from the past."

2. With your next three breaths, let go of all images and thoughts about what you think may happen in the imagined future. Exhale away all the "what if" thoughts. With each exhalation free your muscles, your heart, and your mind of any effort to try to control the so-called future.

Say to yourself as you exhale, "I release my mind and body from the future."

3. With your next three breaths, say, "I choose to be in this present moment, in this place, now. I let go of trying to control any other time or striving to be any other place. I notice

Mourning the Loss, Releasing the Past, Accepting Your Present

Letting go of images of the imagined past or future is a cognitive process of training your brain to access the ease and calm of the present. Mourning the losses and pains of the past, however, is a two-part emotional process of release that involves: one, letting go how little effort it takes to simply breathe comfortably and accept the just right level of energy to focus on this moment and this task—in the only moment there is, now."

Say to yourself as you exhale, "I bring my mind into the present."

4. Tell yourself, "For the next few minutes, there is nothing much for my conscious mind to worry about within this sanctuary of the present. I am safe from the past and the future. I just allow the natural processes of my mind and body to provide me with focused concentration. I easily access the inner genius of my mind and body and its creative resources for recuperation and recovery."

Say to yourself as you exhale, "I am centered within my larger, wiser, stronger Self."

5. With your next three breaths count up from one to three: one, becoming more adequately alert with each breath; two, curious and interested about going rapidly from not-knowing to knowing; and, three, eager to begin, curious and interested about how much I will accomplish in such a short period of time.

You may find it helpful to record this exercise and play it each time you start a project, face a medical procedure, or transition to a new activity or place.

of trying to change what happened; and two, accepting yourself as you are and where you are now. You might think of self-acceptance, therefore, as the positive, flip-side of the mourning process.

Once you stop trying to hold on to the way things were and how you think they should continue to be, your hands and mind are open to accept, work on, and, possibly, enjoy what you have now. This emotional letting go of the past permits you to focus both your mind and your heart on optimizing your chances in the present.

Even if your current situation is unpleasant and difficult, you can make it easier to accept by acknowledging that you are vulnerable to the same problems as any other human being. You might even broaden your compassion for others to include yourself and discover that as you become less self-critical of your current situation, you lower your stress levels. After all, you and your body have been through a lot on your journey of dealing with cancer and life-threatening illness. You've faced one of your worst fears and somehow—with the help of family, friends, counselors, and doctors and nurses—you've lived through it to possibly find that you're less afraid of life's challenges and are more ready than ever to enjoy whatever moments you can.

By letting go of struggling to change the past and by accepting yourself with compassion and understanding, you can expect that you'll make more energy available to improve your health. Even if you don't feel transformed by your experience with cancer, in time you may learn to appreciate the precious moments you have to live more fully.

Shifting Roles

One of my clients, Jean, a thirty-eight-year-old mother of two diagnosed with ovarian cancer, said:

> I feel as if my life has belonged to someone else. What bothers me is not that I might die, but that I never really got to live. Much of my life I lacked confidence and was depressed. But having cancer has taught me to take charge of my decisions and to feel powerful. I want so much to live my life, even if I have only a few months or years.

She then asked me a question that motivated me to write *Awaken Your Strongest Self,* a book about how to live fully without needing a life-threatening wake-up call. Jean asked, "How can I use what I learned from having cancer in my daily life?" She wanted to know how to use the power she gained from taking charge of her cancer treatment and apply it to her family and worklife.

To cope with her cancer, Jean had to shift from her primary roles as a dependable mother, wife, and caretaker to that of a more dependent patient. This shift was uncomfortable for her and her family but necessary if she was going to take care of herself. In our sessions we joked about the familiar announcement made by flight attendants that, in the event of loss of cabin pressure, put the yellow oxygen mask on yourself first before you attempt to assist a child. It serves as a good reminder to those of us who tend to care for others and worry about what they think. At times, we must first take care of ourselves.

Shifting from the role of a provider in the family to being a patient, and then from patient to survivor, can have an unsettling effect on the members of your family as well as your sense of identity. A change in roles can be especially difficult if you base your identity on a job and achievements that may be interrupted by medical conditions and treatments.

Shifting roles, however, can provide another opportunity to transform your life. The impact of cancer can shatter old roles, free you from a limited sense of identity, and leave you open to create a new, truer self. Coping with cancer can motivate you to fashion new rules of life based on your current values and priorities rather than those imposed by society and your past.

Changes in Relationships

Throughout the course of your treatment you most likely will notice that some relationships become deeper, some more superficial, and some may end. When your treatment causes you to appear weak or sick, even some old friends may avoid you, resuming their friendship when you appear healthier. This challenging period of your life will intensify and strengthen whatever relationships remain.

Loving friends and family will do what they can to be supportive of the way you want to fight cancer and of how you want to maintain the quality of your life. You may need to change those relationships which are not supportive of your beliefs and values. But changes in relationships need not be painful or negative. In fact, an honest discussion about your changing roles and perspectives can heighten the quality of healthy relationships.

A supportive family and understanding friends can lessen the solitude of cancer and clarify how important your relationships are to you as you become more fully alive after cancer. Things have changed. You have changed, and with that change comes a new and transformative view of life and of yourself. You may have learned ways of coping with adversity that have caused you to transform into a peak performer with a transformative perspective, a clear focus on the present moment, a release of the past, and freedom from prior roles.

As a result of your challenging journey you have the opportunity to develop the resilience and enhanced coping skills that will improve your life after cancer.

Chapter 10

Coping with End of Life Issues

When further efforts in pursuit of a cure are clearly futile, it's time to take a new direction. In earlier chapters I recommended that patients actively participate in most aspects of their cancer treatment. The same is true for the final stages of life, but with a focus on those activities that add to the quality of the time remaining.

A Change in the Patient's Role

At this point, the patient and family might consider switching from a heroic struggle for a cure to seeking as much comfort as possible. A delay in making this shift in roles may result in the loss of precious time and energy in activities that diminish the quality of the last weeks and days of life.

When facing this difficult decision, it helps if the patient takes the lead in notifying both the family and the doctors that he or she is now aiming for a higher quality of life rather than continuing with the discomfort of more tests and treatments. The transition from fighting for a cure to making the last days comfortable, is made more smoothly when the patient, the family, and the physician are in agreement.

Some patients wish to maintain an active role in their care up to their last days and hours. Yet, many relinquish this role as the end becomes certain, relying on their earlier preparations and their agreements with their family and physician to carry out their wishes.

Just as the cancer patient is more than his or her disease, so too the dying patient is more than a weakening grasp on life. Our society's discomfort with the topic of death leads to the sad fact that in the United States more than 75 percent of those who die each year do so in a hospital or nursing home. This figure includes many who spend their last hours in a sterile and strange environment in which they are subjected to expensive and pointless medical procedures. While modern medical methods can prolong life and lessen pain, they can also complicate the natural process of dying and add to it increased costs, loss of control, and separation from one's family and friends during the last moments of life—a time when patient and family are most in need of contact and communication with each other.

As the National Hospice Organization guidelines state, "When the *quantity* of life is limited, the *quality* of that life must be made optimal."

Preparing for Your Final Days

If your doctor tells you that your cancer is *terminal* or that you are in the terminal stage of cancer, you need to remember that many patients outlive this prognosis by months and even years. In fact, because of the effectiveness of early diagnosis and improved chemotherapy treatments, cancer is now considered a chronic disease. This means that, if cancer is caught early enough, patients usually have time to consider new treatments, to possibly go into remission, and to prepare for their final days.

Regardless of your prognosis, it makes sense to prepare a legal document to help your family cope with your final days and to insure that your wishes about the extent of treatment you receive will be observed. You also will want to decide whether you wish to stop medical treatments such as chemotherapy if they offer minimal hope of remission or cure. Two legal documents—a "Durable Power of Attorney for Healthcare" and a "Living Will"—can minimize the need for your family to argue among themselves and with hospital staff about your wishes. In the Durable Power of Attorney you designate who is allowed to make medical decisions on your behalf should you become unconscious or otherwise incapacitated. It only comes into effect if you are unable to make or communicate responsible decisions concerning your healthcare.

A Living Will, on the other hand, appoints someone to carry out your wishes—regarding suspension of life support or the kind of life-sustaining treatment you wish to receive—if you become incompetent or are in a permanent state of unconsciousness.

When patients are in their last days and are exhausted with treatments and from fighting against a long-term disease, they need a way to tell their family and friends that it's time to let them go. They often express the wish to die at home, free of interference from hospital staff. Several of the cancer patients I've worked with over the last twenty-five years have worried about not knowing how to die and have asked me to help them to let go. I've told them:

> When the time comes, your body will know what to do, and your mind will know how to cooperate with comforting thoughts and feelings. You don't have to continue treatment for your family. If you like, I will help you to tell your family and doctors that you're tired and wish to stop the struggle. I can help you tell them, "Please let me go. I want to stop all treatments and to die in peace at home."

Deciding on Terminal Care

As a patient with a serious condition, you and your family could benefit from knowing that neither illness nor approaching death would diminish the respect, care, and worth accorded you by your healthcare professionals. I would hope that you can rest assured that your wishes will be respected, that any pain would be managed, and that—when the time comes—you will die in peace surrounded by loving family and caregivers. As Dr. Cicely Saunders, founder of hospice care, has stated:

> You matter because you are you. You matter to the last
> moment of your life, and we will do all we can not only
> to help you to die in peace, but also to live until you die.

The hospice movement serves as an excellent model of how to provide care during the last stages of terminal illness. Hospices and home care of the dying now offer patients and families more time together, management of pain, more personal care, and a chance to reduce the financial burden. In many ways this is a break from traditional Western health care that too often considers death as a failure and a departure from the medical mission to save lives. The hospice environment, on the other hand, supports human dignity in death, offering the patient care and comfort rather than aggressive treatment.

There are four main types of terminal care to consider: traditional hospital care, hospice care within a hospital, independent hospice care, and hospice home care.

More information about hospice care is available online at the National Hospice and Palliative Care Organization (NHPCO) website (www.nhpco.org). They can also be reached by mail (1700 Diagonal Road, Suite 625, Alexandria, VA 22314,) by phone (703/837-1500), and by fax (703/837-1233).

Hospice Care for Terminal Patients

Regardless of the current stage of the patient's illness, it's helpful for both the patient and the family to know that hospice care is available if and when it is needed. Also, hospice care can lessen stress and worry of those involved by providing medical professionals who are dedicated to keeping patients comfortable and assisting families throughout the last stages and during bereavement.

Hospice care can provide:

1. Medical treatment that anticipates the patient's pain, thereby keeping the patient virtually pain-free, free of the fear of pain, and alert

2. Symptom relief

3. Home care of the patient (through the use of outpatient care and home visits by nurses and volunteers)

4. Support for the entire family during the patient's illness and with bereavement

5. Comfort knowing that the patient can die at home. (Three out of every four hospice patients in 2006 died in a private residence, nursing home, or other residential facility rather than an acute-care hospital.)

Patients can have as much as 90 percent of their hospice care costs covered by Medicare, private insurance, or Medicaid. Coverage by these plans, however, does require certification by your doctor and the hospice medical director that your condition is terminal with a prognosis of less than six months to live if the illness were to run its natural course.

The initial coverage period is for ninety days and can be re-certified by your physician for an additional ninety-day benefit period followed by an unlimited number of sixty-day periods (each of which requires re-certification by a doctor). This is more than adequate coverage given that average length of service for a patient receiving hospice care is fifty-nine days and often less than twenty-one days.

The Family's Dilemma

The family of a patient with incurable cancer or a life-threatening illness faces several emotional dilemmas that are confounded by imprecise labels such as *terminal* and *dying*. When a patient is given a terminal diagnosis it usually means that his cancer is currently incurable and that the patient is expected to die of that disease within six months. In reality, many so-called *terminal* patients have been known to live ten years or more with their disease. For example, my doctor gave me a terminal diagnosis of less than one year to live. That was over thirty years ago. After surgery and eighteen months of chemotherapy, the diagnosis was changed to cured of any visible cancer.

Another difficulty for the family is that being told that a loved one has a terminal disease can lead to premature mourning while the patient is still very much alive and in need of your visits and presence. A distinction needs to be made between the label *terminal* and the actual process of *dying*—when a patient is in the last days or weeks of his or her life. But no one can know with certainty when a patient will die. If the patient lives for six months, two years, or five years with a so-called *terminal* disease, does that mean that he or she was dying all that time? How much life can be lived in two years, or even six months, if you are not waiting to die?

The medical profession does itself and its patients a disservice when it attempts to make such predictions. Patients and their families need to know that any prediction given by the medical staff is only an opinion, not a fact. For example, the doctors told my family on three occasions that my mother was about to die. Each time she outlived the prognosis by more than a month, surviving months beyond what the doctors predicted. Each time we received the call that our beloved mother was dying we flew and drove to be by her side for what we thought was the last time.

When a medical professional makes such a serious assertion, we assume it's correct. And because we don't want a loved one to die alone, we give voice to that painful thought, "I would never forgive myself if I weren't there when she died."

Hopefully, we can forgive ourselves for being human and, therefore, incapable of curing cancer or of preventing a loved one from dying. We can take comfort, however, in knowing that we did what we could. You might take heart from what Theresa, a nurse, writes in *The New York Times* as she describes her first experience with the sudden death of a patient:

> I did the only thing I could do and you can't say much more than that. What can we do? Go home, love your children, try not to bicker, eat well, walk in the rain,

feel the sun on your face and laugh loud and often, as much as possible, and especially at yourself. Because the antidote to death is not poetry, or drama, or miracle drugs, or a roomful of technical expertise and good intentions. The antidote to death is life.

Pain Control and Symptom Relief

Cancer is so frequently associated with pain that many are surprised to learn that over 50 percent of terminal cancer patients experience negligible pain or none at all. Approximately 10 percent experience only mild or moderate pain and about 40 percent of patients with advanced, terminal cancer have severe pain at some time.

Hospices are especially prepared to head off pain before it starts and to keep patients comfortable. In the hospices and pain clinics, it's understood that physical pain can be relieved once the patient is placed on a regular schedule of medication. With this approach the medication builds in the patient's bloodstream and he or she need never experience pain.

Thus, the "pain-fear-of-pain cycle" is broken, and the patient can be free of the physical tension and psychological stress of anticipating the onset of another bout with pain. Under this system of medication, it's often possible to lower the patient's dosage. And, of course, the patient is not placed in the position of having to experience more pain in order to earn medication, as is often the case when medication is administered on an as needed basis. In addition to using medication to relieve pain, Hospices teach relaxation, biofeedback, and self-hypnosis. While these methods are not for everyone, nor for all types of pain, they can provide patients the feelings of effectiveness and satisfaction that comes with the ability to once again manage one's own body. It's also remarkable for many to learn that physical pain can be relieved without drugging the patient into unconsciousness or a state of grogginess.

Enhancing the Quality of Life

In standard hospital care, the curing function too often supplants the caring function, and when a cure is not likely, we are told the dreadful and false statement, "Nothing more can be done." But, as Dr. Saunders has said so eloquently:

> . . . a time comes when the "healthy" outcome is death and terminal care directed to that outcome is good medicine ... the focus shifts from curing to caring and... the goal is enhancement of the quality of the patient's remaining life, rather than its prolongation.

There can be a remarkable reduction of stress and anxiety for both patient and family when hospice staff shift the focus to medical care and take the focus off struggling for a cure. The wife of a patient at St. Christopher's Hospice in London spoke of the change she noted in herself and her husband when he was transferred from a traditional hospital to the hospice. She said, "I used to dread coming to see him in the other hospital. He was so depressed, in pain, and unable to do much. Now, he eagerly looks forward lo my visits and we're able to go for walks together. It's miraculous what they've done. He's no longer afraid or depressed."

What's so striking about this statement is that, while we continually hope for a miracle cure for cancer, more practical miracles can be achieved among those who cannot be cured of cancer. And symptom relief is often another practical and achievable miracle.

The Patient's Family

A counselor, medical social worker, or chaplain can often help family members of a terminal patient communicate among themselves, with children, and with the patient.

The family and spouse or partner of a dying patient need support in order to cope with their feelings of loss, helplessness, and perhaps, anger and guilt at the patient's leaving them.

Grieving

The death of a loved one is often accompanied by conflicting feelings that are hard to understand. While feelings of sadness and grief are to be expected, you may be surprised to have strong feelings of anger, resentment, fear, and even relief. It's not unusual to have feelings of anger and resentment about the person's leaving, as well as feelings of fear about being alone and lonely and feelings of relief that suffering has come to an end for both you and your loved one.

The grieving process does not take place all at once, but in stages that often must be repeated. It takes time to grasp, both mentally and emotionally, that a loved one is gone and that you are powerless to change that. Grieving is an act of releasing your frustrating struggle to change what's happened and of accepting yourself as human. This act of accepting your human limits is a gift of compassion that stops the frustration of trying to control what's beyond your control and lessens your feelings of guilt.

While it's not easy for the human heart to accept, the truth is that all relationships end with separation or death. The human mind also has difficulty accepting that the comfort of a friend, companion, or lover is lost. Sometimes it requires daily reminders and anniversaries before it acknowledges that something precious has ended. The mind also finds it difficult to let go of trying to solve the problem of how or why something so painful happened. You may need to repeatedly tell yourself, "It's not your fault that you can't prevent these painful losses. You're only human." You may find that counseling, talking with friends, follow-up hospice care, and writing out your feelings are helpful during the process of grieving through the first anniversary of the patient's death.

Guilt

When someone close to us dies we often feel that we could have or should have done something to prevent this death, or said something to ease the suffering. Elisabeth Kübler-Ross, in her book, *On Death and Dying*, suggests that many people find it very difficult to be with a dying patient in the last moments of life yet feel ashamed or guilty if the patient dies alone. One close friend, family member, or nurse can be selected to insure that the someone will be there with the patient in her or his last moments. Thus, all can feel some relief in knowing that the patient will not die alone. And, perhaps more important, the family can be comforted by the knowledge that in the weeks and months during which the patient was still fully conscious, they reached out to provide whatever solace and support they could to a loved one.

Honesty

In almost all cases, both the patient and the family benefit from honest, open talk about the patient's condition. Guarded communication between the family and the medical personnel and futile attempts to hide the truth from the patient can create quite a stressful burden on the family. While it's not necessary to share all your feelings, thoughts, and worries with the patient, it's a time when concealing the truth can leave the patient feeling patronized and isolated.

In contrast, families that are honest can be relaxed and spontaneous and can allow patients to face their condition and choose their own course of action. Once the topics of death and loss are faced openly, the terminal patient can once again be part of the family and be included in the usual topics of conversation. During any crisis—but particularly when a family member is dying—open communication and expression of feelings cement the family into a unit that provides comfort for all its members.

Surprisingly, these last days with a loved one can be very rich. The family often becomes closer by sharing intense feelings and support for each other. This closeness will be especially helpful to the family in weathering the changes and adaptations it will face when reorganizing itself during the days and months of bereavement.

Appendices

A. Exercise for Recall of the Diagnosis
B. Reducing Stress by Making Yourself Safe with You
C. The Patient's Bill of Rights
D. Resources

A. Exercise for Recall of the Diagnosis

In groups I conducted at the University of California Medical Center, the participants found the following exercise beneficial for developing an awareness of their own initial reactions to cancer and their underlying beliefs. This exercise also gave many an opportunity to share, often for the first time, these feelings with those close to them. This exercise is of great help in identifying any troublesome beliefs that persist, unnecessarily taxing your energy and clouding your thoughts.

I suggest that, in preparation for this exercise, you first read it through, setting aside fifteen to thirty minutes to experience the exercise and talk about it with your family. If you do it by yourself, leave time to write down your reactions.

In this exercise we will go back to that time and place when you first heard the diagnosis of cancer for yourself or a loved one.

- Begin by finding a comfortable position, perhaps sitting in a chair with your feet flat on the floor.

- Take three slow, deep breaths, holding your breath briefly, and then exhaling slowly and completely.

- As you exhale, float down into the chair, letting the chair support your body, and let go of muscle tension. Just allow the chair to support your body and the floor to support your feet and legs.

- So now, simply drift back to that time and place when you first were told of the diagnosis. Imagine being in that place: Recreate for yourself that room, the furniture, the colors and lighting, and the sounds and the voices. Just be there and allow your mind to present what it will. Just let it happen.

- Once you are there, back in that place, at that time, focus your attention on three areas within you:

1. Become aware of what you are feeling physically—your muscles, your breathing, your pulse and heartbeat, and anything that makes itself physically evident.

2. Become aware of what thoughts and images are going through your mind, of what you are saying to yourself, and what your attitude is.

3. Become aware of what you are feeling emotionally.

Notice that you can shift from one area of focus to another.

After you've read through the preceding exercise and noted your reactions, return to chapter 2 for a discussion and processing of the experience.

B. Reducing Stress by Making Yourself Safe with You

When you, from the perspective of your compassionate self say the following statements to the frightened and overwhelmed parts of you, you are:

- Sending a message of safety that turns off the stress response

- Transiting to a new, robust self-image that is stronger and wiser than your usual, default, limited identity

- Accessing deep inner resources to cope with changing situations and relationships

- Reducing the stress and anxiety of struggling alone, separated from your True Self

- Empowering yourself to relate to all parts of you from a protective role, a higher perspective, and with a compassionate voice

Note that the following are not the typical positive affirmations. The following regardless statements are more powerful because you are not trying to convince yourself that everything is okay. You get to shift identities by speaking to a small part of yourself—a part that is easily overwhelmed because it acts as if separated from your larger support system. You are then empowered to protect and guide these parts that have limited, outdated ways of coping with life. You, from your new perspective, have an expanded identity that empowers you to protect your body and smaller "egos," by guiding them toward inner peace and safety. In the compassion voice of your adult, protection self, you replace stress with safety and replace separateness with connection by saying:

Regardless of what happens in life, your worth is always safe with me.

[If you prefer, replace "regardless" with "whatever happens," or "no matter what happens."]

Regardless of what you can or cannot do, you are always worthwhile.

Regardless of whether you win or lose, you deserve love, pleasure, and freedom from self-criticism.

Regardless of what happens to you, you deserve to be treated with dignity and respect. I will always respect my life and my body.

Regardless of who stays or who goes, I am on my side. I will never abandon you.

Regardless of how healthy or ill you become, I appreciate the effort, wisdom, and protection given me by you, my body and my spirit.

Regardless of how intense your emotions become, I acknowledge their validity for you, and I accept them completely. I am strong enough to be with your emotions.

Regardless of how uncomfortable others are with you, your feelings or your body, I will always accept you and remain at peace with you.

Regardless of your problems and issues, I accept you and love you completely.

Regardless of the health or weakness of my body, I can always heal my spirit.

C. The Patient's Bill of Rights

(Adapted from the American Cancer Society website, www.cancer.org)

What is the Patient's Bill of Rights?

Following is a summary of the Consumer Bill of Rights and Responsibilities that was adopted by the U.S. Advisory Commission on Consumer Protection and Quality in the Health Care Industry in 1998. It is also known as the Patient's Bill of Rights.

The Patient's Bill of Rights was created with the intent to reach three major goals:

1. To help patients feel more confident in the U.S. health care system, the Bill of Rights:

- assures that the health care system is fair and it works to meet patients' needs

- gives patients a way to address any problems they may have

- encourages patients to take an active role in staying or getting healthy

2. To stress the importance of a strong relationship between patients and their health care providers

3. To stress the key role patients play in staying healthy by laying out rights and responsibilities for all patients and health care providers

This Bill of Rights also applies to the insurance plans offered to federal employees. Many other health insurance plans and facilities have also adopted these values. Even Medicare and Medicaid stand by many of them.

The Eight Key Areas of the Patient's Bill of Rights

1. Information Disclosure

You have the right to accurate and easily-understood information about your health plan, health care professionals, and health care facilities. If you speak another language, have a physical or mental disability, or just don't understand something, help should be given so you can make informed health care decisions.

2. Choice of Providers and Plans

You have the right to choose health care providers who can give you high-quality health care when you need it.

3. Access to Emergency Services

If you have severe pain, an injury, or sudden illness that makes you believe that your health is in serious danger, you have the right to be screened and stabilized using emergency services. You should be able to use these services whenever and wherever you need them, without needing to wait for authorization and without any financial penalty.

4. Participation in Treatment Decisions

You have the right to know your treatment options and take part in decisions about your care. Parents, guardians, family members, or others that you select can represent you if you cannot make your own decisions.

5. Respect and Non-Discrimination

You have a right to considerate, respectful care from your doctors, health plan representatives, and other health care providers that does not discriminate against you.

6. Confidentiality of Health Information

You have the right to talk privately with health care providers and to have your health care information protected. You also have the right to read and copy your own medical record. You have the right to ask that your doctor change your record if it is not correct, relevant, or complete.

7. Complaints and Appeals

You have the right to a fair, fast, and objective review of any complaint you have against your health plan, doctors, hospitals or other health care personnel. This includes complaints about waiting times, operating hours, the actions of health care personnel, and the adequacy of health care facilities.

8. Other Bills of Rights

This bill of rights focuses on hospitals and insurance plans, but there are many others with different focuses. There are special kinds, like the mental health bill of rights, hospice patient's bill of rights, and bills of rights for patients in certain states. Insurance plans sometimes have lists of rights for subscribers. Many of these lists of rights tell you where to go or whom to talk with if you have a problem with your care. The American Hospital Association has a list of rights along with patient responsibilities that can help a person be a more active

D. Resources

American Cancer Society (ACS)

The American Cancer Society has helpful materials that can be ordered from their toll-free number, 1-800-ACS-2345 (1-800-227-2345). A great deal of material is available at the ACS website (www.cancer.org), including information on:

- Medical Insurance and Financial Assistance for the Cancer Patient (also available in Spanish)

- Informed Consent (also available in Spanish)

- Choosing a Doctor and a Hospital (also available in Spanish)

American Hospital Association (AHA)

A brochure from the AHA, The Patient Care Partnership contains information about what patients should expect during their hospital stay and explains their rights and responsibilities. The brochure is available in multiple languages: English, Arabic, Simplified Chinese, Traditional Chinese, Russian, Spanish, Tagalog, and Vietnamese.

It is available as a free download from the AHA website (www.aha.org), in all the languages mentioned above. You can also reach the AHA by phone at 1-800-242-2626.

Centers for Medicare & Medicaid Services

Extensive information is available online (www.cms.hhs.gov/). They can be reached by phone, 1-800-633-4227, or TTY, 1-877-486-2048.

MedlinePlus

MedlinePlus brings together information from the U.S. National Library of Medicine, the National Institutes of Health (NIH), and other government agencies and health-related organizations. Information on patient rights, doctors and dentists, hospitals, clinical trials, Medicare rights, senior long-term care, and more can be found online at www.nlm.nih.gov/medlineplus/patientrights.html

Smokers and Former Smokers

Visit www.smokefree.gov for information and support. Ask your doctor about prescription and over-the-counter drugs that reduce cigarette cravings.

If you are a former smoker, keep in mind that up to half of all lung cancers in the U.S. occur in former smokers. So while your lung health did start to improve the day you quit smoking, a significant cancer risk remains for twenty years or more.

Sisters Network, Inc.

For information on support for black women with cancer see Sisters Network, Inc., a national African-American breast cancer survivorship organization. They can be found online (www.sistersnetworkinc.org), reached by phone, 866-781-1808, or you can send an email to infonet@sistersnetworkinc.org.

Bibliography

Andersen, B. L., Farrar, W. B. Golden-Kreutz, D. M. et al. (2008). "Psychologic Intervention Improves Survival for Breast Cancer Patients: A Randomized Clinical Trial." *Cancer 113*:3450–8.

Andersen, B.L., Farrar, W.B., Golden-Kreutz, D. M., et al. (2007). Distress reduction from a psychological intervention contributes to improved health for cancer patients. *Brain, Behavior, and Immunity. 21*:953-961.

Armitage, C. J., & Conner, M. (2000) ."Social cognition models and health behaviour: A structured review." *Psychology and Health 15*, 173-189.

Borysenko, J. (2007). Minding the Body, Mending the Mind. Da Capo.

Budd, M. (2000). *You Are What You Say: A Harvard Doctor's Six-Step Proven Program for Transforming Stress Through the Power of Language*. New York: Crown.

Burns, D. (1999). *Feeling Good: The New Mood Therapy*. New York: Avon.

Cousins, N. (1981). *Anatomy of an Illness as Perceived by the Patient*. New York: Bantam.

Davey, G.C.L. and McDonald, A.S. (2000). "Cognitive neutralizing strategies and their use across differing stressor types." *Anxiety, Stress, and Coping, 13*,115-141.

Derogatis, L.N., Abeloff, M.D., & Melisaratos, N. (1979). "Psychological coping mechanisms and survival time in metastatic breast cancer." *Journal of the American Medical Association, 242*, 1504-1508.

Derogatis, L.N., Morrow, G.R., Fetting, J., Penman, D., Piasetshy, S., & Schmale, A.M. (1983). "The prevalence of psychiatric disorders among cancer patients." *JAMA, 249*, 751-757.

Endler, N.S. and Parker, J.D.A. (1990). "Multidimensional assessment of coping: A critical evaluation." *Journal of Personality and Social Psychology, 58 ,*844-854.

Fiore, N. A. (2007). *The Now Habit: A Strategic Program for Overcoming Procrastination and Enjoying Guilt-Free Play.* New York: Tarcher/Penguin.

Fiore, N. A. (2006). *Awaken Your Strongest Self: Break Free of Stress, Inner Conflict, and Self-Sabotage.* New York: McGraw-Hill.

Fiore, N. A. (1988). "The Inner Healer." *Journal of Imagery, 12*(2), 79-82.

Fiore, N. A. (1985). Correspondence: "Psychosocial variables and the course of cancer." *New England Journal of Medicine., 313*(21): 1354-1355.

Fiore, N.A. (1984, 1986). *The Road Back to Health: Coping with the Emotional Side of Cancer.* New York: Bantam Books.

Fiore, N. A. (1984). *Healthy Imagining* (Cassette Recording # 301). Berkeley, CA: The Road Back to Health.

Fiore, N.A. (1979). "Fighting cancer—one patient's perspective." *New England Journal of Medicine, 300:*284-9.

Frederick, C. & McNeal, S. (1999). *Inner Strength: Contemporary Psychotherapy and Hypnosis for Ego Strengthening.* Mahwah, NJ: Lawrence Erlbaum.

Garfield, Charles with Bennett, Hal Zina. (1984). *Peak Performance.* Los Angeles: Tarcher.

Goldberg, E. (2001). *The Executive Brain: Frontal Lobes and the Civilized Mind.* Oxford: Oxford University Press.

Gollwitzer, P. M. (1999). "Implementation intentions: Strong effects of simple plans." *American Psychologist, 54,* 493-503.

Harker, B.L. (1972). "Cancer and communication problems: A personal experience." *International Journal of Psychiatry in Medicine, 3,* 163-171.

Holland, J. C. (2001). *The Human Side of Cancer: Living with Hope, Coping with Uncertainty.* Harper.

Kiecolt-Glaser, J. K., Glaser, R., & Williger, D., et al (1985). "Psychosocial enhancement of immunocompetence in a geriatric population." *Health Psychology, 4*(1), 25-41.

Kushner, H. (1983). *When Bad Things Happen to Good People.* New York: Avon.

Lansky, P. (1982). "The Possibility of hypnosis as an aid in cancer therapy."
Perspectives in Biology and Medicine, 25 (3) 496-503.

Larzarus, R. and Folkman, S. (1984). *Stress, Appraisal and Coping.* New York: McGraw-Hill.

Le Doux, J. (1996). *The Emotional Brain,* New York: Simon & Schuster.

Lerner, M. (1996). *Choices In Healing: Integrating The Best of Conventional and Complementary Approaches to Cancer.* MIT Press.

Lippke, S., Ziegelmann, J. P., & Schwarzer, R. (2005). "Stage-specific adoption and maintenance of physical activity: Testing a three-stage model. *Psychology of Sport & Exercise, 6,* 585-603.

Loehr, J., Schwartz, T. (2004). *The Power of Full Engagement: Managing Energy, Not Time, is the Key to High Performance and Personal Renewal.* New York: Free Press.

Luthe, W. (1963). Autogenic Training: Method, research and application in medicine. *American Journal of Psychotherapy, 17,* 174-195.

Luskin, Frederic and Pelletier, Ken R. (2005). *Stress Free for Good: 10 Scientifically Proven Life Skills for Health and Happiness.* HarperOne.

Pelletier, K. R. (1980). *Sound Mind, Sound Body: A New Model For Lifelong Health.* Fireside.

Remen, R. N. (2006). *Kitchen Table Wisdom 10th Anniversary.* Riverhead Trade.

Remen, R. N. (2006). *My Grandfathers Blessings.* Riverhead Trade.

Rosenthal, T. (1973). *How Could I Not Be Among You?* New York: Avon Books.

Rosenthal, T. (1982). "Toxic dumps tied to cancer." *Daily News,* July 9, 1982, p. J1.

Spero, D. (2002). *The Art of Getting Well: Maximizing Health and Wellbeing When You Have a Chronic Illness.* Hunter House.

Taking Time, available from: Office of Cancer Communications, National Cancer Institute, Bethesda, Maryland 20205.

Temoshok, L., Heller, B., Sagebiel, R., Blois, M., Sweet, D., DiClemente, R., & Gold, M. (1985). "The relationship of psychosocial factors to prognostic indicators in cutaneous malignant melanoma." *Journal of Psychosomatic Research, 29*, 139-153.

Trillin, A.S. (1981). "Of dragons and garden peas." *The New England Journal of Medicine*, 304 (12), 699-701.

Weisman, A.D., & Worden, J.W. (1975). "Psychosocial analysis of cancer deaths." *Omega, 6*, 61-75.

Weisman, A.D., Worden, J.W., & Sobel, H.J. (1980). *Psychological screening and intervention with cancer patients* (Final report of the Omega Project, NCI grant #CA-19797). Bethesda, MD: National Cancer Institute.

Weisman, A.D., & Worden, J.W. (1977). "The Existential Plight in Cancer: Significance of the First 100 Days." *International Journal of Psychiatry in Medicine, 7* (1), 1-15.

Index

About the Author

Neil Fiore, Ph.D. is a licensed psychologist in private practice in Berkeley, California; in addition, he coaches internationally. He has served as a psychologist at the University of California at Berkeley, and as a consultant and trainer to business and health institutions. He has appeared on numerous radio and television programs across the country and is widely acknowledged as an expert in the areas of health psychology, optimal performance, stress management, and hypnosis.

He holds a doctorate from the University of Maryland, College Park and a bachelor's degree from St. Peter's College, Jersey City, New Jersey. He served with the 101st Airborne Division in Viet Nam.

31901046999977